Manual on

Sexual and Reproductive Health

An Awakening

AF530752

68th All India Congress of Obstetrics & Gynaecology

aicog Delhi 2026

Advocate Innovate Challenge Optimise Globalise

Manual on
Sexual and Reproductive Health
An Awakening

Series Editors

Ashok Kumar
MD PhD
Director–Professor
Department of Obstetrics and Gynecology
Atal Bihari Vajpayee Institute of Medical Sciences
and Dr Ram Manohar Lohia Hospital
New Delhi, India

Madhavi M Gupta
MS
Director–Professor
Department of Obstetrics and Gynecology
Maulana Azad Medical College and Lok Nayak Hospital
New Delhi, India

K Aparna Sharma
MBBS MD
Professor
Department of Obstetrics and Gynecology
All India Institute of Medical Sciences
New Delhi, India

Editors

Niraj Jadav
Apurba Kumar Dutta
Tripti Sharan

JAYPEE

JAYPEE BROTHERS MEDICAL PUBLISHERS
The Health Sciences Publisher
New Delhi | London

Message from Series Editors

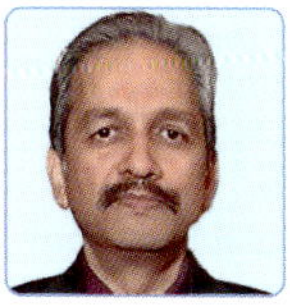

Ashok Kumar
Organizing Chairperson
AICOG-2026
New Delhi

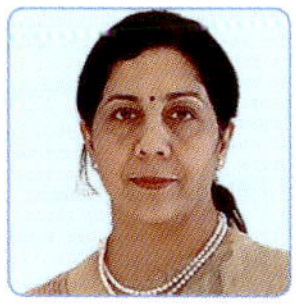

Madhavi M Gupta
Organizing Secretary
AICOG-2026
New Delhi

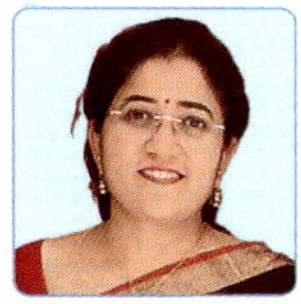

K Aparna Sharma
Organizing Secretary
AICOG-2026
New Delhi

It is after 18 long years that the 68th AICOG is being held in New Delhi. It is a pleasure to welcome you all.

The Organizing Team have poured their heart and soul into curating an academic program which one will feel a loss if missed. The scientific sessions include both national and international faculty who are stalwarts in their fields. There are 18 workshops with 8 full-day and 5 each in the pre-lunch and post-lunch time.

On this occasion, the workshop faculty, have gone that extra mile to publish the workshop manual for eight workshops. This includes all recent scientific evidence and clinical management guidelines. These manuals will serve as a go-to evidence-based resource in your day-to-day clinical practice. We look forward to receiving your valuable feedback.

We acknowledge the hard work put in by all the editors, co-editors, and the authors, who, in spite of busy schedules and time constraints, have contributed immensely.

We would also like to thank M/s Jaypee Brothers Medical Publishers (P) Ltd, New Delhi, India, for partnering with us.

We sincerely hope that you will enjoy reading these manuals, find this manual useful, and treasure it for future use in your practical work.

We take this opportunity to wish you a memorable time during your stay in New Delhi.

Warm Regards

Jaypee Brothers Medical Publishers (P) Ltd

Headquarters
EMCA House, 23/23-B
Ansari Road, Daryaganj
New Delhi 110 002, India
Landline: +91-11-23272143, +91-11-23272703
+91-11-23282021, +91-11-23245672
e-mail: jaypee@jaypeebrothers.com

Corporate Office
4838/24, Ansari Road, Daryaganj
New Delhi 110 002, India
Phone: +91-11-43574357
Fax: +91-11-43574314
e-mail: jaypee@jaypeebrothers.com

Overseas Office
JP Medical Ltd.
83, Victoria Street, London
SW1H 0HW (UK)
Phone: +44-20 3170 8910
e-mail: info@jpmedpub.com

EU GPSR Authorised Representative
Logos Europe, 9 rue Nicolas Poussin
17000, La Rochelle, France
Phone: +33 (0) 6 67 93 73 78
e-mail: contact@logoseurope.eu

Website: www.jaypeebrothers.com
Website: www.jaypeedigital.com

Inquiries for bulk sales may be solicited at: jaypee@jaypeebrothers.com

Manual on Sexual and Reproductive Health: An Awakening

First Edition: **2026**

ISBN: 978-93-7545-939-2

Printed at: Samrat Offset Pvt. Ltd.

Contributors

Aatmik Jain
MBBS Fellow in Psychosexual Medicine
Chief Consultant
Genes Clinic–Infertility and Sexual Rehabilitation Centre
Indore, Madhya Pradesh, India

(Surg Cdr) Deep Kamal
Head
Department of Internal Medicine
Indian Navy, India

Dilpreet Sandhu MBBS MD FICOG
Professor
Department of Obstetrics and Gynecology
Government Medical College and Hospital
Chandigarh, India

Indu Singh MBBS DGO FMAS MICCG
Director
ICGL-Cosmetic Gynecology and Laser Centre
Ujjain, Madhya Pradesh, India

Madhu Kiran MBBS MS
Founder
Kensho Wellness Clinic
Haldwani, Uttarakhand, India

Naisargi Patel
MBBS DGO DNB FICOG CIMP
Consultant
Gayatri Maternity and Nursing Home
Patan, Gujarat, India

Parul Saoji
MS DNB MNAMS FMAS Diploma Cosmetic Gynecology
Cosmetic Gynecologist
Laparoscopic Surgeon and Infertility Specialist
Oracle Clinic
Nagpur, Maharashtra, India

Percy B Kharas MBBS MD DGO FICA (USA)
Chief Consultant
Kharas Hospital
Valsad, Gujarat, India

Reshma Mirge MBBS DGO
Consultant Aesthetic Gynecologist
Sexual Health Consultant
Department of Obstetrics and Gynecology and Sexual Health Medicine and Aesthetic Gynecology
Reeva's Clinic
Pune, Maharashtra, India

Shama Sultana MBBS DGO
Chairwoman and Chief Gynecologist
Hope Win Hospitals
Guntur, Andhra Pradesh, India

Sini S Venugopal
MBBS MD (Obs & Gyne) FMAS DMAS FCLS FICCG FIASRM
Fertility Specialist
Cosmetic and Regenerative Gynecologist
Genix Fertility Care
Bhubaneswar, Odisha, India

Sujoy Dasgupta MBBS MS
Consultant and Clinical Director
Department of Reproductive Medicine
Genome Fertility Centre
Kolkata, West Bengal, India

Swapnita Hota
MBBS DNB FMAS FCLS COSGYN (NACGF, ISARM)
Senior Consultant
Blue Wheel Hospital
Bhubaneswar, Odisha, India

Tripti Sharan
MBBS MS FICOG PGDHHM PGDMLS
Director
Department of Obstetrics and Gynecology
BLK-Max Super Specialty Hospital
New Delhi, India

(Surg Cdr) Vaidehi Thakur MS
Head
Department of Obstetrics
and Gynecology
Indian Navy, India

Vandana Rani Bhuriya MBBS MD
Professor
Department of Obstetrics
and Gynecology
Pt BD Sharma Postgraduate Institute
of Medical Sciences
Rohtak, Haryana, India

Vani Puri MBBS DGO DNB
Senior Consultant
Department of Obstetrics
and Gynecology
Cloudnine Hospital
Ghaziabad, Uttar Pradesh, India

Yogita Gautam MBBS DGO FICOG
Consultant
Department of Obstetrics and
Gynecology
Women's Intimate Health Clinic
Indore, Madhya Pradesh, India

Preface

In a country as diverse and dynamic as India, conversations around sexuality and reproductive health have long-remained shrouded in silence, stigma, and misinformation. Yet, these are not peripheral matters—they lie at the very core of individual well-being, healthy relationships, gender equity, family planning, and the realization of fundamental human rights.

Manual on Sexual and Reproductive Health: An Awakening emerges from a growing recognition that knowledge is the first step toward empowerment, destigmatization, and better health outcomes. This book is both a reflection of and a response to the evolving landscape of sexual medicine in India. It draws inspiration from dedicated workshops and professional gatherings—such as those organized under platforms AICOG—where leading experts come together to share evidence-based insights, clinical experiences, and compassionate approaches to topics that are often avoided in mainstream medical education and public discourse.

From the foundational understanding of the sexual response cycle to the nuanced challenges of female sexual interest/arousal disorder (FSIAD), genitopelvic pain/penetration disorder (including vaginismus), erectile dysfunction, premature ejaculation, menopause and sexuality, sex during pregnancy, and the impact of media on sexual attitudes, this volume covers a broad yet interconnected spectrum. It also addresses critical therapeutic modalities such as Sensate Focus Therapy and Cognitive Behavioral Therapy (CBT), alongside vital sociolegal dimensions including sexual history taking, sexuality across genders, the age of consent in India, and sexual and reproductive rights.

This book is not intended merely as a clinical manual. It is an invitation to awaken—awaken to the reality that sexual and reproductive health is integral to overall health, that shame has no place in healing, and that informed, non-judgmental care can transform lives. Whether you are a healthcare professional seeking to deepen your competence in sexual medicine, a student eager to fill critical gaps in training, a counselor supporting individuals and couples, or simply someone committed to fostering healthier attitudes in society—this text aims to equip you with clarity, sensitivity, and practical wisdom.

We stand at a pivotal moment in India, where increasing awareness, changing social norms, legal advancements, and the courage of both practitioners and individuals are slowly dismantling long-held taboos. May this book serve as a small but meaningful contribution to that collective awakening—one chapter, one conversation, one life at a time.

With gratitude to the efforts of all the editors, co-editors and authors, who have sometimes worked at short notice to submit excellent chapters and articles included in the final publication.

***Editors:* Niraj Jadav, Apurba Kumar Dutta, Tripti Sharan**

Contents

1 CHAPTER

Sexual Response Cycle

Sini S Venugopal

INTRODUCTION

Sexuality is a complex biopsychosocial construct that plays a significant role in the physical health, emotional well-being and interpersonal relationships. In both men and women, sexual functioning is influenced by neuroendocrine regulation, genital physiology, psychosocial dynamics, and cultural context. Although the fundamental components of sexual response are shared across genders, the variability in presentation, hormonal milieu, and life-stage changes requires sensitive and evidence based clinical understanding.

Human sexuality is highly capricious and multifaceted, embracing a composite chemistry of physiologic, psychological and interpersonal components. Though common elements and pathways have been identified, the role of individual differences, learning factors, socio-cultural influences and age on human sexual response cannot be overstated. Human sexual behavior is thus rather complex. In humans, it is the product of complex interactions between both fundamental biological and cultural mechanisms. Despite major advances in understanding the neurobiology of sexual response, defining normal sexual response in both men and women still remains highly challenging and controversial, more so in women.

Health care providers can greatly benefit with a good understanding of the sexual response cycle, which is vital to diagnose sexual dysfunction and to properly provide them with a holistic solution.

William H Masters and Virginia E Johnson in 1966, laid down the first model of human sexual response cycle based on direct observational study **(Table 1 and Figs. 1 and 2)**. They developed one of the foundational models to understand human sexual physiology. It elucidates the complex interplay between neurovascular, endocrine, and psychological mechanisms that govern sexual arousal and satisfaction. Their Linear Model, based on observable physiological changes during sexual activity describes four distinct sequential phases: Excitement, plateau, orgasm, and resolution.

Men usually experience a longer refractory period after orgasm in which they cannot achieve immediate successive orgasms. Women typically have a shorter refractory period, make it possible to have multiple successive orgasms in a row when sexual stimulation continues **(Figs. 3A and B)**.

TABLE 1: Masters and Johnson's linear model of sexual response cycle.

Phase			
Excitement Phase:	Sexual arousal due to physical or psychological stimulation		
	Increase in heart rate, respiration, blood pressure, muscle tone		
	Flushing of the skin		
	Vasocongestion, increased blood flow to genital tissues		
	In men	• Penile erection • Enlargement of the testes • Scrotal tightening	
	In women	• Engorgement of the clitoris, labia majora and minora • Vaginal lubrication	
Plateau Phase:	The excitement phase responses intensifies and stabilize		
	Further increase in heart rate, respiration and blood pressure		
	Muscle tension increases, extend to hands, face, feet and other parts		
	In men	• Testes elevate • Full erection • Pre-ejaculatory fluid secreted at the penile opening	
	In women	• Clitoral glans retracts under the hood • Clitoris becomes increasingly sensitive • Vagina expands • Bartholin's gland produce lubrication in vagina	
Orgasm Phase:	Peak of sexual pleasure with release of sexual tension		
	Shortest phase		
	• Involuntary, rhythmic muscle contractions, more in the muscles of the lower pelvic region (muscles at base of penis/uterus/vagina), but also throughout the body • Feeling of a sense of euphoria		
	In men	Contractions in the muscles at the base of the penis	
		First stage	The vas deferens, seminal vesicles and prostate trigger the urethral bulb to expand with seminal fluid, with internal sphincter contraction closing the bladder neck to prevent urine leakage
		Second stage	Muscles surrounding the base of the penis contract rhythmically, ejaculating semen externally
	In women	Contractions in the uterus and vagina	
Resolution Phase:	Physiological changes return to baseline		
	Muscles relax, blood pressure drops, respiration returns to baseline		
	Blood flow to the genital region decreases		
	Erectile tissues return to normal		

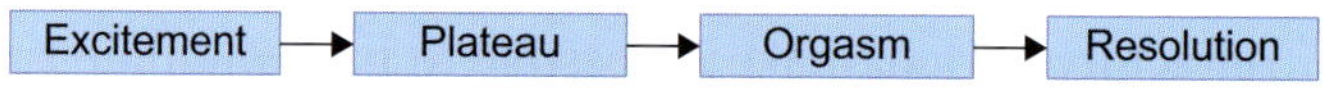

Fig. 1: Masters and Johnson's linear model.

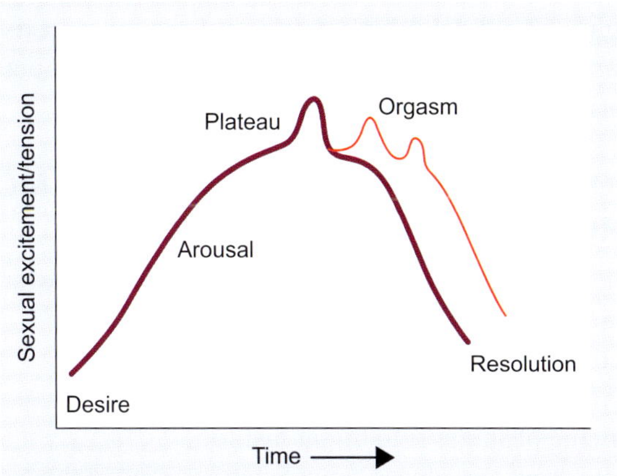

Fig. 2: Masters and Johnson's sexual response cycle.

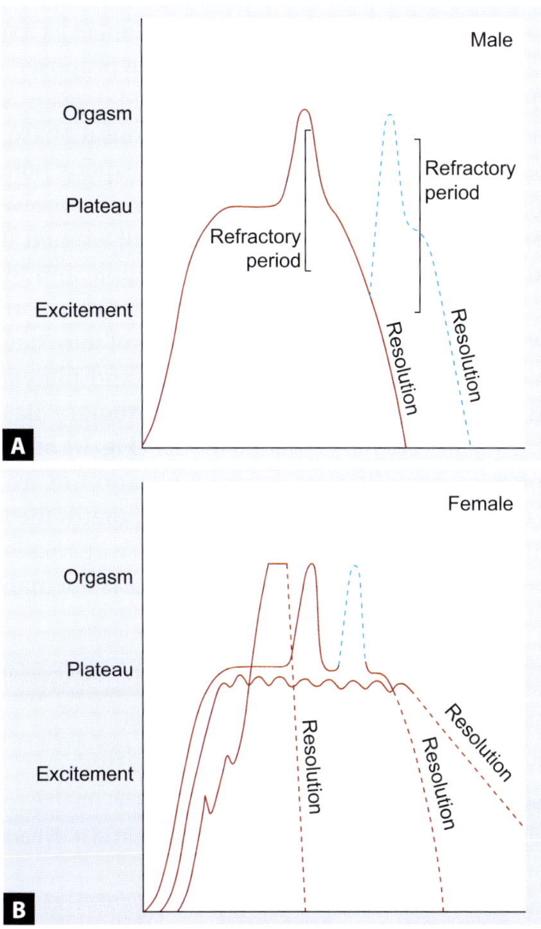

Figs. 3A and B: Refractory period of male and female sexual response cycle.

The traditional sex response cycle has been relatively useful for understanding men's sexual function and dysfunction, but its relevance for women is questionable. However, four fundamental aspects of women's sexuality underlie the need for a different model.

LIMITATIONS OF THE TRADITIONAL LINEAR MODELS OF SEXUAL RESPONSE CYCLE

- It is male biased. It can effectively explain male sexual experience, but not female sexual experience.
- It assumes that sexual desire is a spontaneous drive.
- It assumes that desire and arousal are separate entities.
- The sequencing of stages is in linear fashion.
- It lays emphasis on the physiological components of the sexual response cycle. It considers that the psychological, relational and conceptual aspects are secondary to the physiological aspects of sexual response.

The concept of "desire" was added in 1979 by Kaplan as a separate phase of the human sexual response cycle **(Table 2)**. He proposed the Triphasic Model **(Fig. 4)** consisting of desire, excitement and orgasm. She combined the excitement and plateau stages into a single arousal phase and removed the resolution phase. Still, many sexual medicine experts point out that the process leading from initial arousal to resolution is not always so linear, particularly for women. Upon recognition that all women do not fit into the linear model of sexual response, in 1977 Whipple and Brash-McGreer **(Fig. 5)** suggested a Circular Model of the female sexual response. This concept is based on the Reed's model, consisting of four stages: seduction (encompassing desire), sensations (excitement and plateau), surrender (orgasm), and reflection. Many years later, Rosemary Basson in 2000, suggested a Non-linear Circular Dynamic Model **(Fig. 6)** of sexual response cycle that depicts a very different conceptualization of women's sexual response than the previous linear models. It incorporates the importance of emotional intimacy, sexual stimuli, and satisfaction with relationship **(Figs. 7 and 8)**. Key points include the fact that sexual desire is not mandatory for the

TABLE 2: Evolution of different models of human sexual response cycle.

1966	Masters and Johnson	Linear model
1977	Whipple and Brash- Mc Greer	Circular model
1979	Helen Singer Kaplan	Triphasic linear model
2000	Rosemary basson	Non-linear circular dynamic model

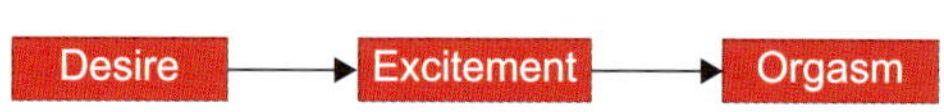

Fig. 4: Kaplan's triphasic model.

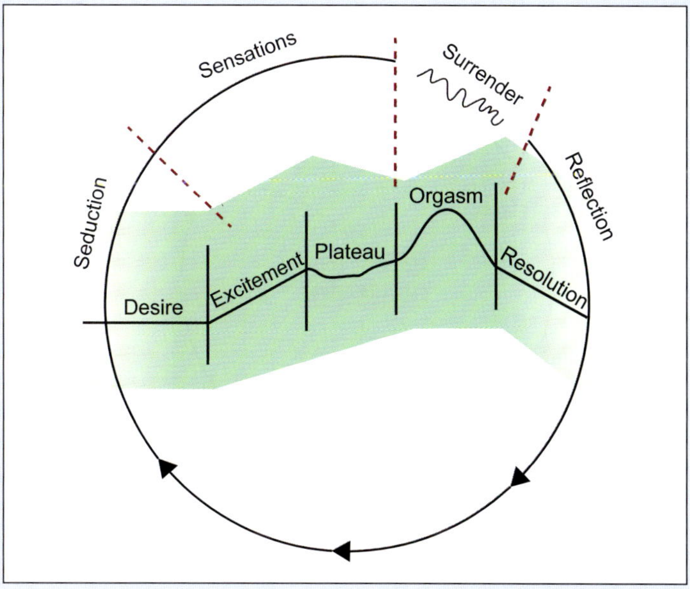

Whipple and Brash-McGreer's circular model of female sexual response shows how pleasure and satisfaction during one sexual experience can lead to the seduction phase of the next sexual experience

Fig. 5: Circular model of female sexual response.

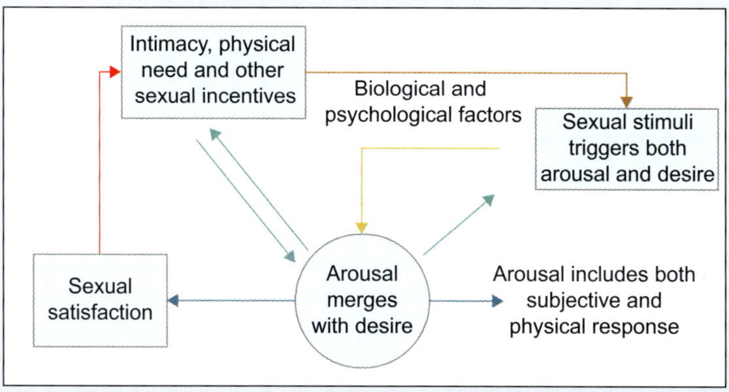

Fig. 6: Non-linear circular dynamic model of sexual response cycle.

sexual response to be initiated, although it might follow pleasurable sexual stimuli **(Table 3)**. The emphasis is on the woman's motivation to engage in sexual activity, and the model is circular, because the positive or negative emotions experienced during each sexual activity will subsequently influence the woman's motivation to engage in subsequent sexual encounters. In fact, female sexual medicine experts believe that many women begin sexual

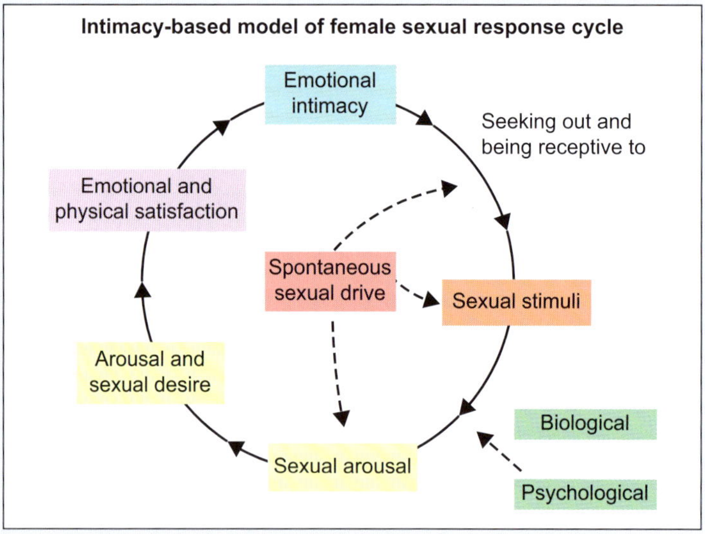

Fig. 7: Role of emotional intimacy in women's sexual response cycle.

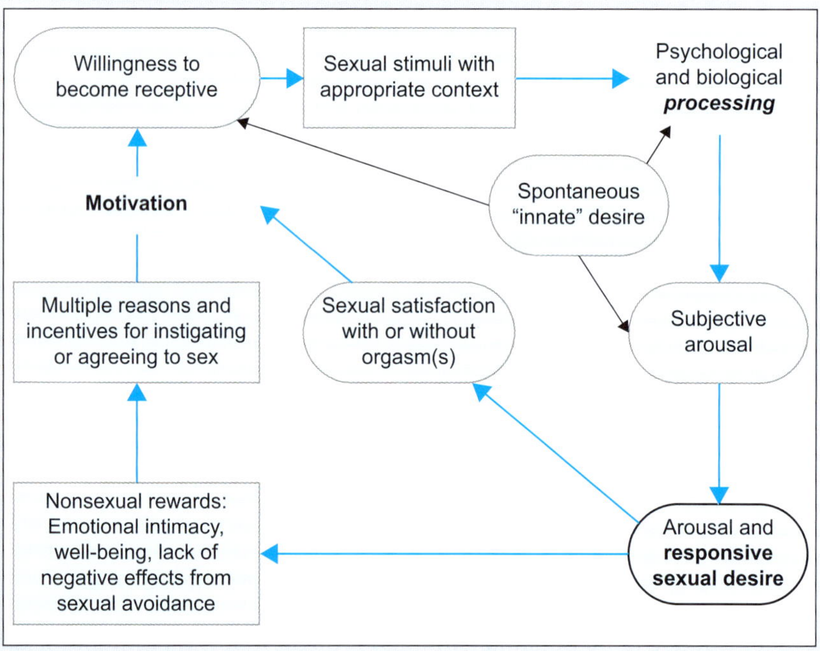

Fig. 8: Role of women's motivation to engage in sexual activity.

activity from a place of sexual neutrality and may experience sexual drive spontaneously at various points throughout the process. This circular model of sexual response acknowledges that orgasms can contribute to satisfaction

TABLE 3: Three main take-home messages regarding human sexual response.

1.	Sexual pleasure and satisfaction aren't reliant on orgasm, though orgasm may certainly be a nice bonus
2.	Sexual desire doesn't always have to precede sexual activity or arousal. Sometimes sexual or non-stimuli, emotional factors, and experiencing arousal will elicit desire
3.	External factors such as relationship dynamics, emotional intimacy, and psychological factors may play an important role in sexual response

but notes that they are not the sole source of pleasure for many women. It also gives more weight to emotional responses and relationship factors in shaping sexual responses, whether positively or negatively.

Understanding the human sexual response cycle is fundamental to recognizing the physiological and psychological processes underlying sexual function and satisfaction. Though, Masters and Johnsons four phase model, remains a cornerstone in sexual medicine, modern perspectives such as Kaplan's triphasic model and Basson's circular model, emphasizes that sexual response is not purely linear, sexual desire and arousal are not always sequential or purely biological phenomena, especially among women. It is influenced by emotional intimacy, cognition, motivation, sociocultural context, relationship dynamics, and individual variability reflecting the multidimensional nature of human sexuality. For clinicians, appreciating this complex interactions is essential for providing empathetic, evidence-based sexual healthcare that respects both biological diversity and human experience.

For clinicians, a nuanced understanding of these evolving concepts is essential for accurate assessment and management of sexual concerns. Today, there is growing recognition that sexuality exists on a wide spectrum, so appreciating similarities, acknowledging differences, integrating biological knowledge with psychosocial awareness and supporting equality in the various dimensions of sexuality, allows for a more holistic and evidence-based understanding of human sexuality—one that honors both the complexity and individuality of the sexual experience to strengthen relationships and promote healthier and more fulfilling emotional lives. Understanding these dimensions helps us approach sexuality with empathy, dignity and scientific awareness.

SUGGESTED READING

1. Journal of Sex &Marital Therapy, 26:1, 51-65, 2000. DOI: 10.1080/009262300278641 Rosemary
2. Rowland, David and Gutierrez, Brittany R., "Phases of the Sexual Response Cycle". Psychology Faculty Publications.2017.62. https://scholar.valpo.edu/psych_fac_pub/62

3. Andersen BL, Cyranowski JM. Women's sexuality: behaviors, responses, and individual differences. J Consult Clin Psychol. 1995;63(6):891-906. doi: 10.1037//0022-006x.63.6.891. PMID: 8543712; PMCID: PMC2707786.
4. Basson R. Human sexual response. Handb Clin Neurol. 2015;130:11-18. doi: 10.1016/B978-0-444-63247-0.00002-X. PMID: 26003236.
5. Rosemary Basson R. The Female Sexual Response Revisited. Journal SOGC. 2000;2(5):378-82. ISSN 0849-5831, https://doi.org/10.1016/S0849-5831(16)30848-5.
6. Basson R. The Female Sexual Response: A Different Model., J Sex Marital Ther. 2000;26(1):51-65.
7. J.R. Georgiadis JR, M.L. Kringelbach ML. The human sexual response cycle: Brain imaging evidence linking sex to other pleasures. Progress in Neurobiol.2012;98(1):49-81. ISSN 0301-0082,2012. https://doi.org/10.1016/j.pneurobio.2012.05.004.
8. Katie R. Giles KR, Marita P. McCabe MP., Original Research—Women's Sexual Health: Conceptualizing Women's Sexual Function: Linear vs. Circular Models of Sexual Response. The Journal of Sexual Med. 2009;6(10):2761-71. ISSN 1743-6095,2009. https://doi.org/10.1111/j.1743-6109.2009.01425.x.
9. Hayes RD, Richard D. "Circular and Linear Modeling of Female Sexual Desire and Arousal. "The Journal of Sex Res. 2011;48(2-3):130-41. Taylor & Francis, Ltd. 2011. http://www.jstor.org/stable/29779463.
10. Leavitt, CE, Leonhardt, ND, Busby, DM. Different Ways to Get There: Evidence of a Variable Female Sexual Response Cycle. The J ournal of Sex Res. 2019;56(7): 899-912. https://www.jstor.org/stable/26778923
11. Masters WH, Johnson VE. Human sexual response. USA: Little, Brown & Co.; 1966.
12. Rosen RC, Barsky JL. Normal sexual response in women. Obstet Gynecol Clin North Am. 2006;33(4):515-26. doi: 10.1016/j.ogc.2006.09.005. PMID: 17116497.
13. Rowland D, Gutierrez BR. (2017). Phases of the Sexual Response Cycle. [online] Available from https://scholar.valpo.edu/cgi/viewcontent.cgi?article=1061&context=psych_fac_pub [Last accessed January, 2026].
14. Toates, F. An Integrative Theoretical Framework for Understanding Sexual Motivation, Arousal, and Behavior. The J ournal of Sex Res. 2009;46(2–3):, 168-93. https://doi.org/10.1080/00224490902747768
15. Wylie K. Masters & Johnson – their unique contribution to sexology. BJ Psych Advances. 2022;28(3):163. doi:10.1192/bja.2021.53

2 CHAPTER

Understanding Female Sexual Dysfunction: Concept and Classification

Yogita Gautam

INTRODUCTION

Sex is one of the most fundamental aspects of human existence, it plays a significant role in women's physical, reproductive, and emotional health. Sexual activity and sexual expression are not limited to reproduction they are also important for emotional health, relationship satisfaction and identity formation. Sex offers several physical emotional and phycological benefits for women. Regular sexual activity enhances emotional bonding, reduce anxiety and stress and self-confidence and body awareness.

WHAT IS SEXUAL HEALTH?

Sexual health as mentioned by the World Health Organization (WHO) refers to "a state of physical, emotional, mental and social wellbeing in relation to sexuality; it is not merely the absence of disease, dysfunction or infirmity".

Sexual dysfunction refers to difficulty that occur during sexual response cycle that prevent the individual from experiencing satisfaction from sexual activity.

Sexual health plays a significant role in women's self-esteem, identity, and relationship satisfaction.

For women sexual health involve:

- A sense of comfort and control over one's body.
- The ability to experience sexual pleasure and intimacy.
- Having sex and consensual sexual relationship
- Freedom from compulsion/force/violence
- Having the right to make choices about sex, contraception, and pregnancy

Benefit or impact of sexual health on women's life:

- Physical health benefits:
    - Reduce stress and anxiety and promote better sleep and immune function.
    - Improve vaginal health and maintain pelvic floor strength.
    - Promote hormonal balance.
- Mental health:
    - Increase self-confidence and body positivity.

    - Support emotional intimacy and connection in relationships.
    - Reduce anxiety and depression.
- Relationship satisfaction:
    - Build trust respect and satisfaction and encourage open communication in relationship.
- Improve overall quality of life and self-esteem and give happiness.

Despite of its significance, female sexual dysfunction (FSD) remains under-recognized, under discussed. Female sexual function and dysfunction is an often-overlooked component within clinical visits.

Sexual dysfunction in women is common yet often remain under-diagnosed due to lack of adequate training and experience of doctor to manage female sexual dysfunctions (FSD).

This lack of education about sexual health, causes myth, mis information and silence about sexual health. This leads to problem in addressing the sexual concerns of patient and leads to misdiagnosed and under diagnosed.

ROLE OF TABOO AND CULTURAL SILENCE

Despite of progress in global health education, the topic of sex and reproduction continue to be surrounded in secrecy, misinformation and stigma.

Due to restriction in society about disclosing sexual health problems lead to chronic stress, anxiety, depression, marital instability and divorce.

If there is a problem such as sexual dysfunction between the couples, they may still live together due to cultural and social conditions; however, they may experience emotional divorce.

It causes delay in diagnosis and contributes to unsafe sexual practices unintended pregnancies and sexually transmitted infections (STI).

FEMALE SEXUAL DYSFUNCTION

Sexual dysfunction in women is common, with a community prevalence of 30 to 50%.

According to DSM-5 (diagnostic and statistical manual of mental disorder 5th edition)

"Sexual dysfunction are heterogenous group of disorder characterized by clinically significant disturbance in person's ability to respond sexually or to experience sexual pleasure."

Key Feature of FSD

- Persistent (lasting > 6 month)
- Causes clinically significant distress
- Not explained by another disorder, medical condition or medication
- May be lifelong or acquired, generalized or situational

Physiological events such as pregnancy, childbirth, menopause, aging as well as gynecological condition like infertility, prolapse, urinary incontinence and gynecological cancer have an impact on sexual wellbeing.

Female sexual dysfunction affects the entire spectrum of ages, races and socioeconomic backgrounds.

The development of clear clinical categories and diagnostic guidelines for FSD are of utmost importance and can be great benefits for clinical and public health uses and disease related research.

Classification of female sexual dysfunction (FSD) provides a structural framework to understand, diagnosis and the management of sexual dysfunction **(Table 1)**.

TABLE 1: DSM-5 classification.

Disorder	*Definition*
Specific to females	
Female orgasmic disorder	Marked delay in, marked infrequency of, or absence of orgasm or markedly reduced intensity of orgasmic sensations experienced on almost all (approximately 75%) or all occasions of sexual activity (in identified situational contexts or, if generalized, all the contexts)
Female sexual interest/ arousal disorder	Lack of, or significantly reduced, sexual interest/arousal in least three of the following: • Absent/reduced interest in sexual activity • Absent/reduced sexual/erotic thoughts or fantasies • No/reduced initiation of sexual activity, and unreceptive to a partner's attempts to initiate • Absent/reduced sexual excitement/pleasure during sexual activity in almost all situations • No/reduced sexual interest in response to any internal or external sexual/erotic cues (e.g., written, verbal, visual) • Absent/reduced genital or nongenital sensations during sexual activity in almost all situations
Genitopelvic pain/ penetration disorder	Persistent or recurrent difficulties with one (or more) of the following: • Vaginal penetration during intercourse • Marked vulvovaginal or pelvic pain during vaginal intercourse or penetration attempts • Marked fear or anxiety about vulvovaginal or pelvic pain in anticipation of, during, or as a result of vaginal penetration • Marked tensing or tightening of the pelvic floor muscles during attempted vaginal penetration

Contd...

Contd...

Disorder	*Definition*
Common to both genders	
Substance/medication induced sexual dysfunction	• Significant sexual dysfunction as per clinical examination • There is evidence from the history, physical examination, or laboratory findings of both • Development of symptoms during or soon after substance intoxication or after consumption or withdrawal of a medication • The same substance or medicine is capable of producing similar symptoms • Those symptoms are not explained by any etiology other than substance/medicine induced • Symptoms presented only after substance/medicine consumption • Symptoms reduce post cessation of the drugs • No sexual comorbidity • The disturbance does not occur exclusively during the course of a delirium. • Significant distress present in the individual • Drugs responsible: – *Antibiotics:* Alter the ecology of the vagina and the vaginal flora, predisposing to inflammation and pain/pruritus – Oral contraceptive pills - lead to hormonal changes predisposing to vulvodynia – Psychotropic medication and antidepressants – reduce libido and arousal – Analgesics – morphine, tramadol – Antihistaminics – cetirizine, loratadine – Cardiovascular drugs – amiodarone, clonidine, digoxin, gemfibrozil, methyl dopa, spironolactone – Miscellaneous – amphetamine, dextroamphetamine, gabapentin, GNRH agonists, indomethacin, ketoconazole, phenytoin, topiramate – *Modified from:* Conaglen HM, Conaglen JV. Drug-induced sexual dysfunction in men and women. Aust Prescr 2013;36:42-5
Other specified sexual disorders	There is distress, but all criteria of above categories are not fulfilled
Unspecified sexual dysfunction	Significant distress occurs, but presentations lack sufficient information to be categorized as a specific diagnosis

CLASSIFICATION OF FEMALE SEXUAL DYSFUNCTION

The latest DSM-5 criteria, classification of FSD include major types being include female orgasmic disorder, female sexual interest/arousal disorders and Genito pelvic pain/penetration disorders.

The most common sexual dysfunction reported were arousal disorder (31.3%) followed by desired disorders (26.8%) orgasm disorders (12.4%).

The international society for the study of women's sexual health (ISSWSH) propose a multi-dimensional, biopsychosocial framework for classifying FSD.

ISSWSH integrate biomedical, psychological and sociocultural perspectives into a biopsychosocial model for female sexual function and dysfunction.

ISSWSH recommends a stepwise diagnostic and management approach integrating medical and psychological and relationship assessment.

The classification of sexual health related conditions was reformulated in 11th revision of International Classification of Diseases (ICD-11) following current evidence, best practice, and taking human rights into consideration, which is expected to reflect and provide guidance for more integrative clinical approaches.

ICD-11 has retained the diagnosis of hypoactive sexual desire dysfunction, which can be applied to both men and women, while the sexual arousal dysfunctions have been classified separately for men and women.

Male and female sexual arousal dysfunctions have been separated in ICD-11. This is a progressive change as female sexual experience is influenced and measured by a multitude of factors related to emotional, physical, and relational aspects as compared to male sexual problems which are more physiological and easily measurable.

In ICD-11, separate categories are provided for men and women (female sexual arousal dysfunction and male erectile dysfunction) to replace ICD-10 category of "failure of genital response," because of anatomical and physiological differences underlying the distinct clinical presentations between men and women.

The ICD-11 category, of orgasmic dysfunction, is gender-neutral and can be applied to both men and women.

EFFECTS AND CONSEQUENCES OF FEMALE SEXUAL DYSFUNCTION (TABLE 2)

Female sexual dysfunction (FSD) has a negative impact on women's quality of life, self-esteem and physical health.

Sexual pain is a common complaint in women of all ages and may include pain in vulva, deep pain with penetration, odd tightening of pelvic musculature.

TABLE 2: Effects and consequences of FSD.

No.	*Domain*	*Effects of FSD*
1	Psychological	Low self-esteem, guilt, frustration, anxiety, depression
2	Emotional/relationship	Reduce intimacy, marital conflict
3	Physical	Vaginal dryness, pain, fatigue in pelvic floor muscle
4	Social	Isolation, reduce confidence, impaired social functioning
5	Quality of life	Over all dissatisfaction, reduce sense of wellbeing, poor sleep and productivity

EFFECTS AND CONSEQUENCE OF FSD

On one hand, mental problems such as depression and anxiety reduce sexual desire and satisfaction; on the other hand, persistent sexual problems can lead to feeling of inadequacy, relational conflicts, and deterioration of mental health.

Sexuality education with full range of bio-psycho-social aspects should be an integral part of the curriculum of all healthcare professionals (including nurses, midwives and physiotherapists).

Build awareness, encourage open communication between partners. Advocate for training for healthcare provider and also address taboo regarding sexual activity. Encourage lifestyle factors that support sexual health (exercise, good general health) since physical and mental health influence mental health function.

By breaking silence around female sexuality and empowering women with knowledge, it is possible to reduce the burden of sexual dysfunction and promote overall wellbeing and quality of life.

KEY POINTS

- Sex is natural, multidimensional human experience that extends beyond reproduction to pleasure, intimacy, bonding and self-expression.
- Sexual health is essential part of overall health. Female sexual dysfunction (FSD) is persistent disturbance in desire, arousal, orgasm or pain that causes significant distress.
- FSD negatively affect mental health, physical health, relationship and quality of life.
- Classification of FSD help in diagnosis, treatment planning and research. It is influenced by biological, social, relational and sociocultural factors.
- The main type of FSD includes FSAID, FOD, GPPPD according to (DSM-5)
- Breaking cultural silence, promoting education, lifestyle modification and integrating sexual health into routine health care can transform women's life.
- FSD represent a sensitive yet significant health issue that deserve equal attention as other physiological and psychological disorder.

SUGGESTED READING

1. Arthur R, Collins M. Female Sexual Dysfunction. Berlin/Heidelberg, Germany: Springer Publishing Company; 2020.
2. Başar K. The Changes in ICD-11 Related to Sexual Health and Dysfunction and Their Implication for Clinical Practice. Turk Psikiyatri Derg. 2025;36:31.
3. Chen CH, Lin YC, Chiu LH, Chu YH, Ruan FF, Liu WM, et al. Female sexual dysfunction: definition, classification, and debates. Taiwan J Obstet Gynecol. 2013;52(1):3-7.
4. Clayton AH, Valladares Juarez EM. Female Sexual Dysfunction. Med Clin North Am. 2019;103(4):681-98.
5. Daneshfar F, Keramat A. Sexual dysfunction and divorce in Iran: A systematic review. J Family Med Prim Care. 2023;12(3):430-9.
6. Dong Y, Zhang L, Lam C, Huang Z. Counteracting sexual and reproductive health misperceptions: Investigating the roles of stigma, misinformation exposure, and information overload. Patient Educ Couns. 2024;120:108098.
7. Erdős C, Kelemen O, Pócs D, Horváth E, Dudás N, Papp A, et al. Female Sexual Dysfunction in Association with Sexual History, Sexual Abuse and Satisfaction: A Cross-Sectional Study in Hungary. J Clin Med. 2023;12(3):1112.
8. Gianotten WL, Alley JC, Diamond LM. The Health Benefits of Sexual Expression. Int J Sex Health. 2021;33(4):478-93.
9. Kaundal A, Renjhen P, Kumari R, Jha RP, Marwaha PD, Kaur H, et al. Female sexual dysfunction-knowledge, attitude, practices, and barriers encountered by medical fraternity across the country: A web-based cross-sectional study. J Family Med Prim Care. 2024;13(4):1284-90.
10. Krakowsky Y, Grober ED. A practical guide to female sexual dysfunction: An evidence-based review for physicians in Canada. Can Urol Assoc J. 2018;12(6):211-6.
11. Parameshwaran S, Chandra PS. The New Avatar of Female Sexual Dysfunction in ICD-11—Will It Herald a Better Future? J Psychosex Health. 2019;1(2):111-3.
12. Phillips NA, Bachmann G. Female sexual dysfunction. In: Bieber EJ, Sanfilippo JS, Horowitz IR, Shafi MI (Eds). Clinical Gynecology. Cambridge: Cambridge University Press; 2015. pp. 75-84.
13. Prabhu SS, Hegde S, Sareen S. Female sexual dysfunction: A potential minefield. Indian J Sex Transm Dis AIDS. 2022;43(2):128-34.
14. Razki K, Larnaout A, Najar C, Ben Aissa S, Lansari R, Melki W. Breaking the Taboo: Unveiling the Prevalence and Predictors of Female Sexual Dysfunction in Tunisia. European Psychiatry. 2024;67(S1):S768.
15. Roytman MV, Barnett RL, Rubin RS. Female Sexual Function and Dysfunction. Obstet Gynecol. 2025;146(5):645-59.
16. Srivastava R, Thakar R, Sultan A. Female sexual dysfunction in obstetrics and gynecology. Obstet Gynecol Surv. 2008;63(8):527-37.
17. Vasconcelos P, Carrito ML, Quinta-Gomes AL, Patrão AL, Nóbrega CA, Costa PA, et al. Associations between sexual health and well-being: a systematic review. Bull World Health Organ. 2024;102(12):873-887D.

3 CHAPTER

Female Sexual Interest and Arousal Disorders

Dilpreet Sandhu

INTRODUCTION

Female sexual dysfunctions (FSDs) are broadly classified into three specific categories: female sexual interest/arousal disorder, genitopelvic pain/penetration disorder, and female orgasmic disorder. Estimates of sexual dysfunction prevalence vary widely for both sexes, with 10–52% of men and 25–63% of women reported having one or more sexual related dysfunctions.

In PRESIDE study, 43.1% US women were found to be affected by sexual problems. Sexual distress was reported in 12.0% of respondents, more common in women aged 45–64 years (14.8%) than in younger (10.8%) or older (8.9%) women. A study in four EU countries showed that increase in female sexual dysfunction (FSD), particularly loss of sexual desire, is directly correlated with increasing age. However, the distress associated with loss of sexual desire is inversely correlated with age. WISHeS found the prevalence of HSDD ranged from 9% in naturally postmenopausal women to 26% in younger surgically postmenopausal women. The prevalence of HSDD was significantly greater among surgically postmenopausal women, aged 20 to 49 years, than premenopausal women of similar age, whereas there were no significant differences in the prevalence between surgically postmenopausal women, aged 50 to 70 years, and naturally postmenopausal women. For many women, HSDD was associated with emotional and psychological distress as well as significantly lower sexual and partner satisfaction.

FSIAD a combination of hypoactive sexual desire disorder and female sexual arousal disorder, formerly defined as 2 separate disorders in the *Diagnostic and Statistical Manual of Mental Disorders, Fourth Edition, Text Revision* (*DSM-IV-TR*). Due to the link between sexual desire, interest, and physical arousal, both entities were reclassified as the singular condition FSIAD in *DSM-V* **(Table 1)**.

Diagnosing Female Sexual Interest/Arousal Disorder

To diagnose FSIAD, 3 of the following 6 symptoms must be present for at least 6 months and need to be causing clinically significant distress:

1. Absent or reduced interest in sexual activity
2. Absent or reduced sexual or erotic thoughts or fantasies
3. Absent or reduced initiation of sexual activity and typically unreceptive to a partner's attempts to initiate sex

TABLE 1: DSM classification of FSIAD.

DSM-IV- Diagnoses (2000)	*Changes in DSM-5 (2013)*
Female hypoactive desire disorder	Female sexual interest/arousal disorder (FSIAD)
Female arousal disorder	
Female orgasmic disorder	Same
Dyspareunia	Genito-pelvic pain/penetration disorder
Vaginismus	

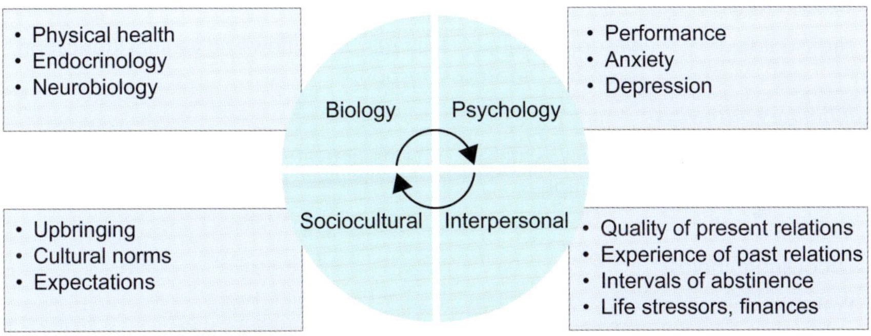

Fig. 1: Biopsychosocial model of female sexual desire.

4. Absent or reduced sexual excitement or pleasure during sexual activity in all or almost all, between 75 and 100%, of sexual encounters (in identified situational contexts if limited to specific situations or in all contexts if generalized)
5. Absent or reduced sexual interest or arousal in response to any internal or external sexual or erotic stimuli or cues
6. Absent or reduced genital or nongenital sensations during sexual activity in almost all or all, between 75 and 100%, sexual encounters (with this being identified as situational if limited to specific contexts or in all contexts if generalized)

ETIOLOGY

Female sexuality is controlled by complex interactions among physiological, psychological, anatomical, neurochemical, hormonal, pharmacological, and social factors. Biopsychosocial Model explains woman's desire for sex and sexual response **(Fig. 1)**. It integrates all of the components which can serve as a basis for understanding HSDD.

Physiologically, sexual desire involves hormone status, energy metabolism, autonomic arousal in the hypothalamus, and the intensity of the stimuli that prime the attention in the hypothalamus and limbic system. Excitatory and inhibitory neurochemical systems control sexual response

TABLE 2: Neurotransmitters and hormones: Important role in sexual desire.

Excitatory pathways	
Dopamine	Positively influences pleasure/ reward pathways in the brain
Norepinephrine	Important for sexual desire and motivation, elevated during sexual arousal and orgasm
Melanocortins	
Oxytocin	
Estrogen Testosterone	Act centrally and peripherally to promote desire and arousal, facilitate blood flow and vaginal lubrication
Nitric Oxide	Vasodilator effect facilitates blood flow and vaginal lubrication, promote the arousal response
Inhibitory pathways	
Serotonin	Restrict excitatory systems, activated during periods of sexual inhibition
Opioids	
Endocannabinoids	
Prolactin	
Progesterone	

and are activated or suppressed by steroid hormones and experience-driven changes in gene expression and neurochemical function.

A key issue concerns the neurotransmitters involved in the control of genital sexual arousal **(Table 2)**. At the peripheral level, acetylcholine plays a role in the regulation of vaginal blood flow and vaginal smooth muscle contractions. Vasoactive intestinal peptide and nitric oxide are responsible for the increase in vaginal blood flow during sexual arousal, whereas noradrenaline is likely inhibitory. In the central nervous system, serotoninergic projections from the brain to the spinal cord likely inhibit the induction of genital arousal by peripheral information.

Sexual dysfunction often has a large impact on quality of life. HSDD was also associated with significant decrements in general health status, including aspects of mental and physical health.

Barriers to diagnosis: Women often do not themselves mention these issues to the healthcare providers. A survey on 450 women with self-reported low sexual desire, showed that 73% of premenopausal women and 81% of postmenopausal women reported having never mentioned their desire problems to a health care provider. In another larger survey, only 34.5% of 3,239 women with a distressing sexual problem had formally discussed their problems with their health care providers. Hence, embarrassment largely contributes to women's unwillingness to seek help from a health care provider. A survey completed by 1,196 women who sought routine Pap smear screening at a clinic showed that, for at least 45% of patients, the topic of sexual health was not raised during their visit. However, most of these women (~85%) expressed that the topic would be easier to discuss if the provider broached the topic, which indicates an untapped opportunity for improved communication and care.

Gynecologic cancer survivors often hesitate to raise sexual health concerns with their clinicians. A pilot test Starting the Conversation (STC) showed that 35% and 45% of women raised or asked about sexual health concerns during the post-intervention clinic visit, respectively, versus 0 and 27% in the control arm. Data support the STC intervention as feasible and acceptable, with promising effects for gynecologic cancer survivors' communication about sexual health concerns.

The healthcare practitioners rarely inquire about any sexual problems due to various reasons including limited time with patients, discomfort with the topic, and a perceived lack of effective therapies. Screening for HSDD can be accomplished in a time-efficient manner during an office visit. Decreased sexual desire screener (DSDS) is a five item self-reported questionnaire, a validated tool to assist in the diagnosis of acquired, generalized HSDD **(Table 3)**.

TABLE 3: Decreased sexual desire screener (DSDS).

1	In the past, was your level of sexual desire or interest good and satisfying to you?	☐ Yes	☐ No
2	Has there been a decrease in your level of sexual desire or interest?	☐ Yes	☐ No
3	Are you bothered by your decreased level of sexual desire or interest?	☐ Yes	☐ No
4	Would you like your level of sexual desire or interest to increase?	☐ Yes	☐ No
5	Please mark all the factors that you feel may be contributing to your current decrease in sexual desire or interest:	☐ Yes	☐ No
A	An operation, depression, injuries, or other medical condition	☐ Yes	☐ No
B	Medications, drugs, or alcohol you are currently taking	☐ Yes	☐ No
C	Pregnancy, recent childbirth, or menopausal symptoms	☐ Yes	☐ No
D	Other sexual issues you may be having (pain, decreased arousal, or orgasm)	☐ Yes	☐ No
E	Your partner's sexual problems	☐ Yes	☐ No
F	Dissatisfaction with your relationship or partner	☐ Yes	☐ No
G	Stress or fatigue	☐ Yes	☐ No

Female Sexual Function Index (FSFI): A validated19-item questionnaire that assesses the main dimensions of sexual function: desire, arousal, lubrication, orgasm, global satisfaction, and pain. The desire domain (FSFI-d) assesses the frequency and degree of desire. The Female Sexual Distress Scale- Revised (FSDS-R) is a questionnaire that allows the measurement of distress related to sexual dysfunction and specifically low desire using item13 (FSDS-R-13).

Evaluation of FSIAD case: Recognize underlying conditions contribute to the reduced desire.

- Major relationship or physical issues.
- *Soliciting more detailed information of low desire:* onset, duration, behavioral adaptation and avoidance, and level of distress.
- *Complete gynecologic history:* Any sexually transmitted diseases, History of sexual abuse, Urinary or bowel complaints, and/or prior surgery
- Close evaluation of the patient's
  - Medical history (including reproductive history),
  - Comorbid conditions (endocrine, neurologic, cardiovascular, and psychiatric disorders),
  - Use of prescription and over-the-counter medications **(Table 4)**
- *Psychiatric disorders:* Depression and anxiety, should be considered in the differential diagnosis as potential contributing factors to low desire.
- Targeted physical examination (as indicated)
- Specific tests based on patient history and physical examination, such as physical findings suggestive of thyroid disease or hyper-prolactinemia.

TABLE 4: Drugs adversely affecting sexual desire.

Drug class	*Medications*
Antiepileptic drugs	Carbamazepine, phenytoin, primidone
Cardiovascular and antihypertensive agents	ACE inhibitors, amiodarone, β-blockers (atenolol, metoprolol, propranolol), calcium channel blockers, clonidine, digoxin, diuretics (hydrochlorothiazide, spironolactone), lipid-lowering agents
Hormonal medications	Antiandrogens (flutamide), GnRH agonists, oral contraceptive pills
Pain relievers	NSAIDs, opiates
Psychotropic medications	Prolactin-inducing antipsychotics, anxiolytics (alprazolam, diazepam), lithium, SNRIs, SSRIs, tricyclic antidepressants
Other	Chemotherapeutic agents, histamine receptor blockers, indomethacin, ketoconazole
Drugs of abuse	Alcohol, amphetamines, cocaine, heroin, marijuana

TREATMENT

As FSIAD etiology has various aspects hence a holistic approach should be adopted, comprising of initial office-based counselling to address basic sex education, clarify common myths and misconceptions, make general changes in behavior and lifestyle to improve sexual interest and intimacy. If problem does not improve then next step is the PLISSIT (Permission, Limited Information, Specific Suggestions, Intensive Therapy) model, an incremental approach to office-based counselling.

If the office-based counseling is found insufficient or if, the history of trauma, abuse, or serious psychiatric issues is detected, then referral to psychotherapist is the next step. Psychotherapy interventions starts with addressing the cognitive aspects to modify thoughts, beliefs, behaviors, emotions and relationship issues that interfere with desire.

Mindfulness training: It involves cultivating non-judgmental awareness of the present moment, encouraging participants to connect with and engage in their sexuality through learning and practicing a range of mindfulness exercises. These exercises aim to enhance present-moment awareness, acceptance, and self-compassion.

Couple Therapy

- *Cognitive behavior therapy:* It serves to change sexual behavior by focusing on pleasure and self-exploration instead of planned sexual activity or avoidance of sexual activity.
- *Sensate Focus Therapy:* A technique introduced by the Masters and Johnson. It works by refocusing the participants on their own sensory perceptions and sensuality, instead of goal-oriented behavior focused on the genitals and penetrative sex.
- Use of erotic materials (if acceptable to the patient).

The Female Sexual Function Index (FSFI) has been used in randomized controlled clinical trials to assess the outcome. Drugs predisposing to FSIAD should be modified or changed.

Pharmacotherapy

Flibanserin: FDA approved for the treatment 48 of acquired, generalized HSDD in premenopausal women, at a daily dose 100-mg tablet at bedtime. It decreases serotonin levels and increases dopamine and norepinephrine levels, work on brain function by enhancing excitatory elements and lessening the inhibitory response to sexual cues. Most common adverse effects are dizziness, somnolence, nausea, fatigue, insomnia, and dry mouth. These risks are increased when combined with alcohol or cytochrome P450 3A4 (CYP3A4) inhibitors (e.g., fluconazole). Flibanserin ingestion should be delayed by at least 2 hours after alcohol ingestion; patients who consume three or more alcoholic beverages are advised to skip their evening flibanserin dose.

Bremelanotide: A melanocortin receptor agonist, approved by the FDA in June 2019 for treatment of HSDD in premenopausal patients, administered as a subcutaneous injection (1.25 and 1.75 mg), through an auto-injector ≥ 45 minutes prior to anticipated sexual activity, should not use >8 doses per month. The most common adverse events include nausea (40%), vomiting (5%), flushing (20%), and headache (11%) and hyperpigmentation (1%). It is found to be teratogenic in animal studies, so effective contraception use is recommended.

Testosterone: A recent systematic review and meta-analysis included 7 randomized controlled studies, composed of more than 3,000 postmenopausal women treated with the transdermal testosterone patch shows significant increases in sexual desire, sexual activity, SSE, and orgasms and a significant decrease in personal distress compared with women in the placebo group. 0.5 gm of 1% cream or 5 mg gel applied daily. Oral testosterone intake is associated with adverse changes in liver function and lipids. FDA did not approve a testosterone transdermal patch usage due to paucity of long-term safety data.

Topical vaginal estrogen: first-line therapy for vulvovaginal atrophy, the available evidence does not support the use of systemic estrogen therapy for female sexual dysfunction (e.g., HSDD).

Bupropion: FDA approved to treat depression and assist with smoking cessation; use for sexual dysfunction, including that induced by SSRIs, is an off-label indication. 12-hour and 24-hour extended-release formulations, started as 150 orally once daily dose in morning for 2–4 weeks and observed for increased anxiety, insomnia and hypertension.; then increase to 300 mg once daily if needed.

Bupropion plus trazodone: In studies of patients with major depressive disorder, a lower incidence of sexual dysfunction was observed for bupropion, a dopamine and norepinephrine reuptake inhibitor, compared with other agents. The combination of bupropion plus trazodone acts to increase dopamine and norepinephrine and modulate serotonin and found to be effective in premenopausal women with HSDD.

Sildenafil: Phosphodiesterase (PDE-5) inhibitor, 50–100 mg orally, not more than once a day, 1–4 hours prior to sexual activity, improves genital arousal in women. Side effects include headache, flushing and nausea. It is contraindicated in patients taking nitrates.

Sublingual testosterone plus sildenafil, a phosphodiesterase type 5 inhibitor: improves sexual desire and genital arousal. The most common treatment-related adverse events associated with testosterone plus sildenafil were flushing (23.0%) and headache (15.9%).

Sublingual testosterone with buspirone: which is a serotonin 1A receptor agonist with immediate short-term decreases in serotonergic activity, improved sexual functioning in women with HSDD and over-activation of sexual inhibitory mechanisms. Common adverse events included dizziness (11.3%) and light headedness (10.3%).

Neuromodulation therapy: The use of electrical stimulation to modulate neural circuit activity, currently not FDA-approved for sexual dysfunction, however therapies designed for bladder or bowel dysfunction have been shown to often benefit sexual function.

Herbal supplements: Use should be avoided as the safety and efficacy of these products is unproven. May cause serious side effects due to minimal regulatory oversight.

TAKE HOME MESSAGES

- FSIAD is a type of female sexual disorder with quite high prevalence.
- It has great impact on the quality of life, both physical and psychological.
- It can be primary or secondary, generalized or situational.
- Detailed history taking including sexual history, interpersonal relations, drug intake, physical examination to look for organic underlying cause and lab tests are recommended for the etiology.
- Management starts with office-based counselling then stepping forward to psychotherapy and pharmacotherapy.

SUGGESTED READING

1. Abdolrasulnia M, Shewchuk RM, Roepke N. Management of female sexual problems: perceived barriers, practice patterns, and confidence among primary care physicians and gynecologists. J Sex Med. 2010;7:2499-508.
2. Adebisi OY, Carlson K. Female Sexual Interest and Arousal Disorder. In: StatPearls. Treasure Island (FL): Jan 2025.
3. Annon JS. Behavioral treatment of sexual problems: brief therapy. Hagerstown, MD: Harper & Row; 1976.
4. Balon R. Burden of sexual dysfunction. J Sex Marital Ther. 2017;43:49-55.
5. Basson, R. (2003). Biopsychosocial models of women's sexual response: applications to management of 'desire disorders.' Sexual and Relationship Therapy. 2003;18(1):107-15.
6. Tim M. Bruns TM, Lauren Zimmerman Hershey LZ. Neuromodulation for the treatment of sexual dysfunction: An opportunity for the field. Current Opinion in Biomedical Engineering. 2024;32:100564.
7. Buster JE. Managing female sexual dysfunction. Fertil Steril. 2013;100:905-15.

8. Clayton A, Goldfischer E, Goldstein I, DeRogatis L, Nappi R, Lewis-D'Agostino DJ, et al. Validity of the decreased sexual desire screener for diagnosing hypoactive sexual desire disorder. J Sex & Marital Ther. 2009;39:132-43.
9. Clayton AH, Kingsberg SA, Goldstein I. Evaluation and Management of Hypoactive Sexual Desire Disorder. Sex Med. 2018;6(2):59-74.
10. Harry A. Croft HA. Understanding the Role of Serotonin in Female Hypoactive Sexual Desire Disorder and Treatment Options. The Journal of Sexual Medicine. 2017;14(12):1575-84.
11. Dooley EM, Miller MK, Clayton AH. Flibanserin: from bench to bedside. Sex Med Rev. 2017;5:461-9.
12. Giuliano F, Rampin O, Allard J. Neurophysiology and pharmacology of female genital sexual response. J Sex Marital Ther. 2002;28 Suppl 1:101-21.
13. Graziottin A. Prevalence and evaluation of sexual health problems—HSDD in Europe. J Sex Med. 2007;4 Suppl 3:211-9.
14. Grotas A, Marissa K. "Sexual dysfunction." Sexual and Reproductive Health: A Practical Guide for Primary Care. Cham: Springer International Publishing;, 2022. pp. 163-75.
15. https://www.fda.gov/news-events/press-announcements/fda-approves-new-treatment-hypoactive-sexual-desire-disorder-premenopausal-women
16. Ishak WW, Waguih William and Gabriel Tobia G. "DSM-5 Changes in Diagnostic Criteria of Sexual Dysfunctions." Reproductive System and Sexual Disord. 2013;ers 2(2013):1-3.
17. Kingsberg SA, Woodard T. Female sexual dysfunction: focus on low desire. Obstet Gynecol. 2015;125:477-86.
18. Kingsberg SA. Attitudinal survey of women living with low sexual desire. J Womens Health (Larchmt). 2014;23:817-23.
19. Leiblum SR, Koochaki PE, Rodenberg CA, Barton IP, Rosen RC. Hypoactive sexual desire disorder in postmenopausal women: US results from the Women's International Study of Health and Sexuality (WISHeS). Menopause. 2006;13(1):46-56.
20. Nusbaum MR, Helton MR, Ray N. The changing nature of women's sexual health concerns through the midlife years. Maturitas. 2004;49:283-91.
21. Pfaus JG. Pathways of sexual desire. J Sex Med. 2009;6:1506-33.
22. Reese JB, Bober SL, Sorice KA, Handorf E, Chu CS, Middleton D, et al. Starting the Conversation: randomized pilot trial of an intervention to promote effective clinical communication about sexual health for gynecologic cancer survivors. J Cancer Surviv. 2024;18(3):800-9.
23. Rosen R, Brown C, Heiman J, Leiblum S, Meston C, Shabsigh R, et al. The Female Sexual Function Index (FSFI): a multidimensional self-report instrument for the assessment of female sexual function. J Sex Marital Ther. 2000;26:191-208.
24. Segraves RT, Clayton A, Croft H, Wolf A, Warnock J, et al. Bupropion sustained release for the treatment of hypoactive sexual desire disorder in premenopausal women. J Clin Psychopharmacol. 2004;24:339-42.
25. Shifren JL, Johannes CB, Monz BU. Help-seeking behavior of women with self-reported distressing sexual problems. J Womens Health (Larchmt). 2009;18:461-8.
26. Shifren JL, Monz BU, Russo PA, Segreti A, Johannes CB. Sexual problems and distress in United States women: prevalence and correlates. Obstet Gynecol. 2008;112(5):970-8.

4 CHAPTER

Female Orgasmic Disorder

Reshma Mirge

DEFINITION

Female orgasmic disorder (FOD) is a sexual dysfunction characterized by a persistent or recurrent delay, infrequency, or absence of orgasm following a normal sexual excitement phase, or markedly reduced intensity of orgasmic sensations, causing personal distress or interpersonal difficulty.

The condition is defined in the DSM-5 as "marked delay in, infrequency of, or absence of orgasm, or markedly reduced intensity of orgasmic sensations, on almost all (75–100%) occasions of sexual activity for a minimum duration of 6 months."

Definition and nomenclature of Female orgasmic disorder laid down by International Society for the Study of Women's Sexual Health sexual disorders, including level of evidence.

Female orgasm disorders (Grade = B, level of evidence = 2–3)

Characterized by a persistent or recurrent distressing compromise of orgasm frequency, intensity, timing, and/or pleasure associated with sexual activity for/more than 6 months.

- *Frequency:* Orgasm occurs with decreased frequency (diminished frequency of orgasm) or is absent (anorgasmia)
- *Intensity:* Orgasm occurs with less intensity (muted orgasm).
- *Timing:* Orgasm occurs too late (delayed orgasm) or too soon (spontaneous or premature orgasm) than desired by the woman
- *Pleasure:* Orgasm occurs with absent or decreased pleasure (anhedonic orgasm, pleasure dissociative orgasm disorder) (expert opinion)

EPIDEMIOLOGY

- Prevalence rates vary widely from *10 to 40%* among women, depending on definitions and cultural contexts.
- Lifetime prevalence is higher than point prevalence, as many women experience transient orgasmic difficulty.
- It is more commonly reported in younger women, those with inadequate sexual education, or those with unsatisfactory relationships.

ETIOLOGY

The causes of Female Orgasmic Disorder are *multifactorial*, involving a dynamic interplay between biological, psychological, interpersonal, and sociocultural influences. A clear understanding of these dimensions is essential for accurate diagnosis and effective management.

Biological Factors

These factors contribute to disruption of the *neurovascular and hormonal mechanisms* that mediate arousal and orgasmic response.

- *Hormonal Deficiencies:* Low levels of estrogen and testosterone can impair vaginal lubrication, genital sensitivity, and sexual responsiveness. Estrogen deficiency (common in menopause or surgical oophorectomy) may lead to vaginal atrophy, while low testosterone can reduce sexual energy and intensity of orgasmic sensations.
- *Neurological Disorders:* Any lesion affecting the spinal cord or peripheral nerves (such as diabetic neuropathy or multiple sclerosis) can interfere with the transmission of sensory impulses from the genitalia to the brain, diminishing orgasmic capacity.
- *Pelvic Surgery or Childbirth Trauma:* Episiotomy scars, pelvic floor injury, or post-surgical nerve damage (after hysterectomy or prolapse repair) may alter genital sensation and produce anxiety about sexual activity.
- *Chronic Illnesses:* Conditions like diabetes mellitus and hypertension impair vascular and neural function, leading to decreased genital engorgement and sensitivity. Chronic pain syndromes also divert focus from sexual pleasure.
- *Medications:* Selective Serotonin Reuptake Inhibitors (SSRIs), antipsychotics, antihypertensives, and oral contraceptives are well-known to delay or inhibit orgasm by altering central neurotransmitter pathways, especially serotonin and dopamine.

Psychological Factors

Psychological elements play a *pivotal role*, as orgasm is not merely a physical reflex but a psychophysiological experience requiring emotional surrender and mental engagement.

- *Anxiety, Guilt, or Fear:* Anticipatory anxiety or guilt about sex—often rooted in moral or cultural conditioning—can inhibit arousal and block orgasmic release.
- *Past Sexual Trauma or Abuse:* Traumatic experiences may create subconscious fear, avoidance, or dissociative responses during intimacy.
- *Depression and Low Self-Esteem:* Depressive states suppress libido and emotional responsiveness; women with poor self-image may feel undeserving of pleasure.

- *Performance Anxiety and Relationship Discord:* Fear of failure or partner criticism can prevent relaxation, which is essential for orgasm. Constant self-monitoring disrupts spontaneous sexual flow.

Sociocultural Factors

Society and upbringing exert profound influence on women's sexual expression.

- *Restrictive Sexual Upbringing:* Environments that equate sexuality with shame or sin discourage exploration and body awareness, fostering guilt around pleasure.
- *Lack of Sexual Education:* Inadequate knowledge about female anatomy and arousal pathways leaves many women unaware of their own sexual response potential.
- *Gender Role Conditioning and Body Image Issues:* Unrealistic beauty standards or patriarchal expectations can create self-consciousness and anxiety, inhibiting sexual freedom.
- *Myths Regarding Female Sexuality:* Beliefs such as "good women should not enjoy sex" or that orgasm must occur through penetration alone can cause unnecessary distress and feelings of inadequacy.

Interpersonal Factors

Since orgasmic response is highly dependent on *trust, intimacy, and communication*, relational dynamics are often decisive in determining sexual satisfaction.

- *Poor Communication with Partner:* Lack of openness about desires, preferences, or dissatisfaction can perpetuate misunderstanding and mechanical sexual interactions.
- *Lack of Trust or Emotional Intimacy:* Emotional distance reduces psychological safety, preventing relaxation necessary for orgasm.
- *Partner's Sexual Problems:* Partner's premature ejaculation, erectile dysfunction, or low libido can indirectly reduce stimulation and emotional engagement, resulting in secondary orgasmic difficulty.

The multi factorial causes of female orgasmic disorder are summarized in **Table 1**.

PATHOPHYSIOLOGY

The orgasmic response in females represents a highly integrated neurovascular and psychosexual event, involving complex coordination between the central nervous system (CNS), autonomic pathways, and peripheral genital sensory feedback.

During sexual stimulation, afferent sensory signals from the genitalia and erogenous zones are transmitted via the pudendal, hypogastric, and

TABLE 1: Etiological factors in female orgasmic disorder.

Domain	*Contributing factors*	*Underlying mechanisms/effects*
Biological	Hormonal deficiencies, neuropathy, chronic illness, surgery, drugs	Reduced genital sensitivity, impaired neurovascular response
Psychological	Anxiety, guilt, trauma, depression, low self-esteem	Inhibits relaxation, increases performance anxiety
Socio Cultural	Myths, restrictive upbringing, body image issues	Guilt and ignorance about pleasure
Inter personal	Communication gaps, partner dysfunction	Emotional disconnect, inadequate stimulation

pelvic nerves to the spinal cord and further relayed to higher cortical and subcortical centers, primarily the limbic system (amygdala, hippocampus), hypothalamus, and nucleus accumbens.

Activation of these regions triggers emotional arousal, pleasure perception, and autonomic outflow leading to orgasmic release.

At the neurochemical level, dopamine, oxytocin, norepinephrine, and melanocortins facilitate sexual excitation and orgasm, whereas serotonin and prolactin exert inhibitory effects. Optimal dopaminergic and oxytocinergic signaling within the mesolimbic reward pathway is essential for sexual satisfaction and climax. Dysregulation of these neurotransmitters—due to medications (such as SSRIs), endocrine changes, or mood disorders—can attenuate sexual responsiveness and delay or abolish orgasm.

The hypothalamus, especially the medial preoptic area (MPOA) and paraventricular nucleus (PVN), plays a pivotal role by integrating hormonal cues (estrogen, testosterone, oxytocin) with neural signals to modulate genital vasocongestion, muscle contraction, and rhythmic discharges characteristic of orgasm.

Peripheral vascular responses involving nitric oxide (NO)-mediated vasodilation contribute to clitoral engorgement and vaginal lubrication—both prerequisites for orgasmic potential.

Flowchart 1 shows the neurohormonal axis pathway that leads to the female orgasm. It also shows sites of dysfunction.

In *Female Orgasmic Disorder*, pathophysiological mechanisms may involve:

- *Central dysregulation* of limbic or hypothalamic circuits resulting in impaired dopaminergic drive or oxytocin release.
- *Peripheral neuropathic damage* (e.g., diabetic neuropathy, spinal cord injury, pelvic surgery) that interrupts sensory feedback pathways.
- *Hormonal deficiencies*, particularly reduced estrogen and testosterone, leading to diminished genital sensitivity and vascular response.

Flowchart 1: The neurohormonal axis pathway that leads to the female orgasm.

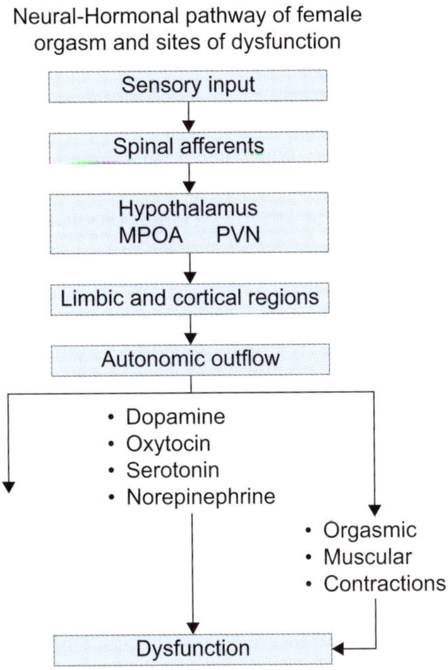

- *Psychological inhibition* stemming from anxiety, trauma, or relationship distress, which activates the cortical network and suppress limbic arousal.

Thus, orgasmic dysfunction seldom arises from a single cause; it reflects a *multifactorial disruption* involving neuroendocrine imbalance, psychogenic inhibition, and interpersonal disharmony.

Female Orgasmic Disorder can be classified into four major types based on onset and situational variability **(Table 2)**.

DIAGNOSTIC CRITERIA AND EVALUATION

DSM-5-TR Diagnostic Criteria for Female Orgasmic Disorder

Female Orgasmic Disorder is defined as a *persistent or recurrent delay in, infrequency of, or absence of orgasm*, or *markedly reduced intensity of orgasmic sensations* following a normal sexual excitement phase.

The diagnosis requires that:

1. *Symptoms have persisted for a minimum duration of 6 months,*
2. *Cause clinically significant distress* to the individual, and
3. *Cannot be better explained* by:
   - A nonsexual mental disorder,
   - Severe relationship distress,
   - Other significant stressors, or
   - Effects of a substance, medication, or another medical condition.

TABLE 2: Classification of female orgasmic disorder.

Type	*Definition*	*Description and clinical implications*
Primary (Lifelong)	The woman has never experienced orgasm under any circumstances—whether during intercourse, masturbation, or other sexual activities	Often linked to *developmental, educational, or psychosexual factors* such as restrictive upbringing, lack of sexual knowledge, or deep-seated psychological inhibition. Anatomical or neurological causes should also be ruled out
Secondary (Acquired)	The woman has previously achieved orgasm, but has become unable to do so	Usually associated with *biological, psychological, or relational changes,* including menopause, medical illness, medication use (e.g., SSRIs), trauma, or relationship stress. This type often responds well to psychosexual therapy once the precipitating factor is identified
Situational (Most Common)	The woman experiences orgasm only in specific situations or forms of stimulation, such as masturbation or oral sex, but not during vaginal intercourse	Suggests *context-specific psychological or relational barriers.* Common causes include inadequate stimulation, performance anxiety, or lack of communication with the partner
Generalized	The woman is unable to experience orgasm in all situations, regardless of the type of stimulation or partner	Indicates a more *global dysfunction,* often involving *neuroendocrine, psychological, or severe interpersonal issues.* Comprehensive evaluation is essential to determine underlying factors

DSM-5-TR Symptom Criteria

At least one of the following must be present in *most sexual encounters (75–100%)*:

- Marked delay in, infrequency of, or absence of orgasm.
- Markedly reduced intensity of orgasmic sensations.

Specifiers

Specifier	*Description*
Lifelong vs. Acquired	Whether the difficulty has been present since the beginning of sexual life or developed after a period of normal function
Generalized vs. Situational	Whether the dysfunction occurs in all settings or only under specific circumstances (e.g., with one partner or type of stimulation)
Severity	Mild, Moderate, or Severe, depending on the degree of distress and functional impairment

CLINICAL EVALUATION

A detailed, *biopsychosocial assessment* is essential to differentiate between organic and psychogenic causes and to plan appropriate therapy.

History Taking

- *Sexual history:* Onset, duration, frequency, situational triggers, type of stimulation, satisfaction level.
- *Medical history:* Chronic illnesses (diabetes, hypertension, neurological disorders), hormonal status, obstetric and gynecological history.
- *Medication history:* Antidepressants (SSRIs), antipsychotics, anti-hypertensives, oral contraceptives.
- *Psychological factors:* Anxiety, depression, trauma, guilt, or relationship stress.
- *Sociocultural influences:* Sexual education, upbringing, cultural taboos, myths about female sexuality.

Physical Examination

- *General examination:* Secondary sexual characteristics, signs of endocrine dysfunction.
- *Pelvic examination:* Sensation, muscle tone, signs of atrophy, pain, or scarring (if indicated).
- *Neurological assessment:* Reflexes, perineal sensitivity, and spinal integrity if neuropathy is suspected.

Laboratory and Imaging Workup (if Indicated)

- Serum *estrogen, testosterone, prolactin, and thyroid function tests.*
- *Blood glucose levels* for diabetic neuropathy screening.
- *Pelvic ultrasonography* or *MRI* in suspected structural or postoperative cases.

Psychological and Relationship Assessment

- Explore *emotional intimacy, communication patterns, and partner response.*
- Use validated tools such as the *Female Sexual Function Index (FSFI)* or *Sexual Distress Scale (SDS)* for quantification.
- Involve the partner during counseling to assess relational dynamics.

Various differential diagnosis can be taken into consideration as illustrated in **Table 3.**

A structured diagnostic approach to female orgasmic disorder is outlined in **Flowchart 2.**

TABLE 3: Differential diagnosis for female orgasmic disorder.

Condition	*Distinguishing features*
Female Sexual Interest/Arousal Disorder	Lack of desire or arousal precedes difficulty with orgasm.
Genito-Pelvic Pain/Penetration Disorder	Pain or fear of penetration overshadows orgasmic concerns.
Medication-Induced Sexual Dysfunction	Temporal relation to drug initiation (e.g., SSRIs, antihypertensives).
Endocrine Disorders (Hypoestrogenism, Hypothyroidism)	Associated systemic or menstrual symptoms, confirmed by labs.

Flowchart 2: Diagnostic evaluation of female orgasmic disorder.

Patient with orgasmic difficulty
↓
Detailed sexual and medical history
↓
Physical and neurological examination
↓
Identify biological factors (Hormonal, neurological, drug-related)
↓
Assess psychological and interpersonal components
↓
Rule out other sexual dysfunctions (Arousal, pain)
↓
Integrate findings → Diagnosis → Tailored management plan

MANAGEMENT OF FEMALE ORGASMIC DISORDER

The management of Female Orgasmic Disorder (FOD) requires an *individualized, multidimensional approach*, integrating *psychological, behavioral, pharmacological, and relational strategies*. The primary goal is to restore sexual satisfaction, enhance emotional intimacy, and address distress associated with orgasmic dysfunction.

Psychoeducation

- Psychoeducation forms the foundation of therapy.
- Patients are educated about the normal variability in sexual response and the anatomy and physiology of orgasm.
- Myths regarding female sexuality and orgasm (e.g., that orgasm must occur with penetration) are corrected.
- Emphasis is placed on communication, relaxation, and self-acceptance, helping reduce shame, guilt, or fear linked to sexuality.
- Visual aids or diagrams of genital anatomy may be used to improve self-awareness.

TABLE 4: Various methods, techniques and therapeutic targets of behavioral therapy.

Technique	*Therapeutic aim*
Sensate Focus Exercises	Developed by Masters and Johnson; involves non-demand touching between partners to rebuild sensual connection and reduce performance pressure. Focuses on touch, texture, and temperature rather than goal-oriented intercourse
Directed Masturbation Training	Encourages women to explore their own bodies using visual, tactile, and mental stimulation to understand individual arousal triggers. Often combined with guided imagery or vibratory stimulation
Communication and Feedback Training	Enhances emotional closeness and allows partners to express preferences, feedback, and reassurance—key in overcoming situational or relational barriers

Behavioral Therapy

Behavioral interventions focus on *reducing anxiety*, *enhancing body awareness*, and *retraining sexual response* through graduated exercises **(Table 4)**.

Cognitive–Behavioral Therapy (CBT)

- CBT addresses *negative thought patterns* associated with guilt, trauma, or body image concerns.
- Helps restructure maladaptive beliefs such as "I must please my partner" or "I'm inadequate."
- Promotes positive self-talk, emotional regulation, and mindfulness during sexual experiences.
- Particularly beneficial in women with *secondary FOD* following trauma or relational distress.

Pharmacologic Therapy

Pharmacologic interventions are considered when *biological or medication-induced causes* are identified. Evidence remains limited, and pharmacotherapy is best used *adjunctively with psychotherapy* **(Table 5)**.

Physical and Sensory Interventions

- *Pelvic Floor Muscle Training (Kegel Exercises):* Enhances awareness of pelvic sensations, strengthens muscle tone, and improves orgasmic intensity.
- *Vibratory Stimulation:* Provides mechanical sensory input, particularly helpful in women with decreased genital sensitivity or after pelvic surgery.

TABLE 5: Mechanism of actions of various drugs that can be used to treat female orgasmic disorder.

Drug and approach	*Mechanism*
Bupropion	A norepinephrine–dopamine reuptake inhibitor that enhances dopaminergic activity, thereby improving sexual desire and orgasmic response
Sildenafil (PDE-5 inhibitor)	Promotes genital vasocongestion and clitoral blood flow; some benefit reported in SSRI-induced FOD, though data remain limited
Tibolone/Hormone Replacement Therapy (HRT)	Restores estrogen and testosterone balance in peri- or postmenopausal women, improving genital sensitivity and lubrication
Drug Adjustment	For SSRI-induced orgasmic delay, consider dose reduction, drug holiday, or switch to *bupropion* or *mirtazapine* with lower sexual side-effect profile

TABLE 6: Various therapies available and its mechanism of action in details.

Therapy	*Mechanism/evidence*
Mindfulness-Based Sexual Therapy (MBST)	Combines meditation and sensory awareness to reduce anxiety, enhance body connection, and improve orgasmic focus. Demonstrated efficacy in clinical trials
Neurovascular Regenerative Therapy (Experimental)	Involves low-intensity shockwave or exosome-based approaches aiming to restore neurovascular integrity in genital tissue; promising but requires further research
Couple Therapy	Focuses on shared understanding, empathy, and restoration of emotional intimacy within the sexual relationship

- *Biofeedback Therapy:* Teaches voluntary control of genital muscle contraction, reinforcing sexual confidence.

Emerging and Adjunctive Therapies (Table 6)

Flowchart 3 shows the management of Female Orgasmic Disorder (FOD) that requires an individualized, multidimensional approach, integrating psychological, behavioral, pharmacological, and relational strategies.

PROGNOSIS

Most women with Female Orgasmic Disorder (FOD) show a favorable outcome when treatment combines psychosexual therapy, behavioral retraining, and partner involvement.

Improvement rates of 70–80% are reported with regular participation in therapy and good partner communication.

Prognosis depends on the underlying cause, duration of symptoms, and psychological resilience.

Flowchart 3: Stepwise management of female orgasmic disorder.

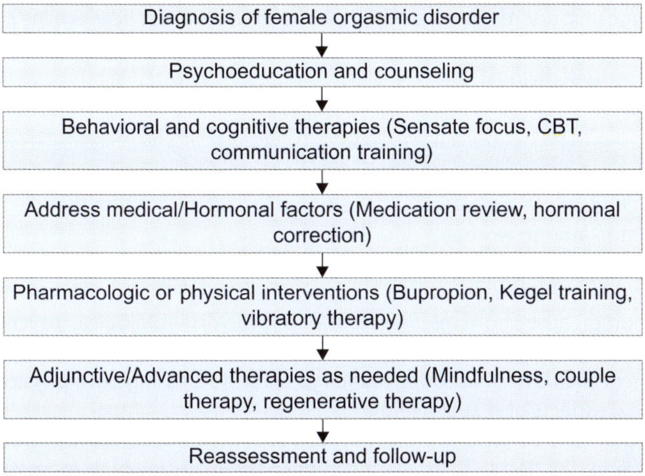

TABLE 7: Prognostic factors in female orgasmic disorder.

Favorable factors	*Unfavorable factors*
Supportive and communicative partner	Relationship conflict or neglect
Secondary or situational dysfunction	Lifelong or generalized dysfunction
Early therapy initiation	Delayed or inconsistent therapy
Absence of psychiatric illness	Comorbid anxiety/depression
Motivation and follow-up adherence	Poor insight or low compliance

Flowchart 4: Determinants of prognosis in female orgasmic disorder.

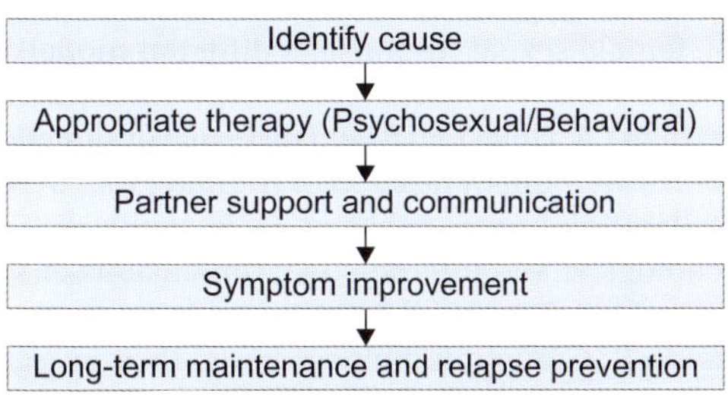

Secondary or situational FOD usually responds better than lifelong forms. Women who receive early counselling, sexual education, and supportive relationships maintain long-term benefits, whereas chronic medical or psychological issues may delay recovery.

Key prognostic determinants influencing treatment outcomes are outlined in **Table 7**.

The determinants influencing long-term outcomes and relapse prevention are illustrated in **Flowchart 4**.

MESSAGE BOX

"Female orgasmic disorder is not a flaw, but a gentle disconnect between the body, mind, and emotions. Healing begins with awareness, empathy, and a guided rediscovery of one's own sensual rhythm."

KEY POINTS

- *Female Orgasmic Disorder (FOD)* is a common yet often under-recognized sexual dysfunction among women.
- It is characterized by a *persistent delay, infrequency, or absence of orgasm* that leads to personal or relational distress.
- The condition arises from *multiple contributing factors*—biological, psychological, interpersonal, and sociocultural.
- *Assessment should be holistic and nonjudgmental*, addressing both physical and emotional aspects of sexual health.
- *Psychosexual and behavioral therapies*, such as sensate focus, cognitive-behavioral therapy, and directed self-stimulation, remain the mainstay of treatment.
- *Pharmacological and hormonal interventions* serve as supportive measures when indicated.
- *Involvement of the partner* fosters mutual understanding and improves therapeutic outcomes.
- A *compassionate, informed, and open clinician–patient dialogue* is fundamental to successful management and long-term recovery.

SUGGESTED READING

1. American Psychiatric Association. Diagnostic and Statistical Manual of Mental Disorders, 5th edition, Text Revision (DSM-5-TR). Washington DC: American Psychiatric Publishing; 2022.
2. Bancroft J, Graham CA. The varied nature of women's sexuality: unresolved issues and a theoretical approach. Horm Behav. 2011;59(5):717-29.
3. Basson R. The female sexual response: a different model. J Sex Marital Ther. 2000;26(1):51-65.
4. Berman JR, Berman LA, Goldstein I. Female sexual dysfunction: new treatments, new opportunities. Int J Impot Res. 1999;11(Suppl 1):S205-12.
5. Brotto LA, Atallah S, Johnson-Agbakwu C, Rosenbaum T, Abdo CHN, Byers ES, et al. Psychological and interpersonal dimensions of sexual function and dysfunction. J Sex Med. 2016;13(4):538-71.
6. Brotto LA, Basson R. Group mindfulness-based therapy significantly improves sexual desire in women. J Sex Med. 2014;11(11):2785-94.
7. Brotto LA, Klein C. Psychological treatments for female sexual dysfunction: state of the evidence. J Sex Med. 2010;7(1 Pt 2):383-401.
8. Brotto LA, Seal BN, Rellini AH. Pilot study of a brief mindfulness-based cognitive behavioral intervention for women with sexual distress and low sexual desire. Sex Marital Ther. 2012;38(4):317-36.
9. Clayton AH, Hamilton DV. Female sexual dysfunction. Psychiatr Clin North Am. 2010;33(4):673-89.
10. Clayton AH, Juarez EM, Goldfischer ER, Hackett G. Evaluation of the female sexual function index (FSFI): cross-cultural applicability. J Sex Med. 2014;11(12):2935-43.

11. Clayton AH, Kingsberg SA, Goldstein I. Evaluation and management of hypoactive sexual desire disorder. J Sex Med. 2018;15(12):1770-82.
12. Faubion SS, Rullo JE. Updates on female sexual dysfunction: diagnosis and treatment. Mayo Clin Proc. 2015;90(5):698-702.
13. Kaplan HS. The New Sex Therapy: Active Treatment of Sexual Dysfunctions. New York: Brunner/Mazel; 1974.
14. Kingsberg SA, Althof SE. Evaluation and treatment of female sexual disorders: an overview. Int J Clin Pract. 2009;63(8):1158-68.
15. Kingsberg SA, Clayton AH, Pfaus JG. The female sexual response: contemporary models and pharmacological management of dysfunction. J Sex Med. 2019;16(4):596-610.
16. Levin RJ. The physiology of sexual arousal in the human female: a recreational and procreational synthesis. Arch Sex Behav. 2002;31(5):405-11.
17. Lorenz TA, Harte CB, Hamilton LD, Meston CM. Evidence for a curvilinear relationship between sympathetic activity and women's sexual arousal. Psychophysiology. 2012;49(1):111-7.
18. Masters WH, Johnson VE. Human Sexual Response. Boston: Little, Brown & Co.; 1966.
19. McCabe MP, Sharlip ID, Lewis R, Atalla E, Balon R, Fisher AD, et al. Incidence and prevalence of sexual dysfunction in women and men: a consensus statement. J Sex Med. 2016;13(2):144-52.
20. Meston CM, Hull E, Levin RJ, Sipski M. Disorders of orgasm in women. J Sex Med. 2004;1(1):66-8.
21. Nappi RE, Cucinella L. Advances in pharmacotherapy for female sexual dysfunction. Expert Opin Pharmacother. 2021;22(2):223-33.
22. Nappi RE, Salonia A, Traish AM, van Lunsen RH, Vignozzi L, Simon JA. Clinical evaluation of testosterone in women: current status and future directions. Sex Med Rev. 2022;10(2):288-303.
23. Parish SJ, Goldstein AT, Goldstein SW, Goldstein I, Pfaus JG, Clayton AH, et al. Toward a more evidence-based nosology and nomenclature for female sexual dysfunctions: updated definitions and classifications from ISSWSH. Sex Med. 2019;7(3):329-42.
24. Segraves RT, Balon R. Sexual dysfunction in women: treatment strategies. World J Psychiatry. 2014;4(2):58-70.
25. Shifren JL, Monz BU, Russo PA, Segreti A, Johannes CB. Sexual problems and distress in United States women: prevalence and correlates. Obstet Gynecol. 2008;112(5):970-8.

5 CHAPTER

Vaginismus: An Underrated Yet Important Intimate Issue

Indu Singh

INTRODUCTION

Vaginismus is defined—according to DSM-IV-TR—as "recurrent or persistent involuntary spasm of the musculature of the outer third of the vagina which interferes with coitus and causes distress and interpersonal difficulty."

This sexual disorder has a significant impact on young women and couples and is a predisposing factor for anxiety disorders. According to the definition, involuntary spasm of musculature is an important requirement for the diagnosis of vaginismus. In one study, only 28% of the vaginismus group had vaginal muscle spasms, and only 24% had pain during attempted sexual intercourse.

It has been classified as

- *Primary:* when the woman has never experienced non painful penetrative sexual intercourse.
- *Secondary:* when she has experienced non painful penetrative intercourse in the past.

  Vaginismus is comorbid with dyspareunia.

PATHOPHYSIOLOGY

The fear avoidance model of pain is often used to conceptualize the development of vaginismus **(Fig. 1)**.

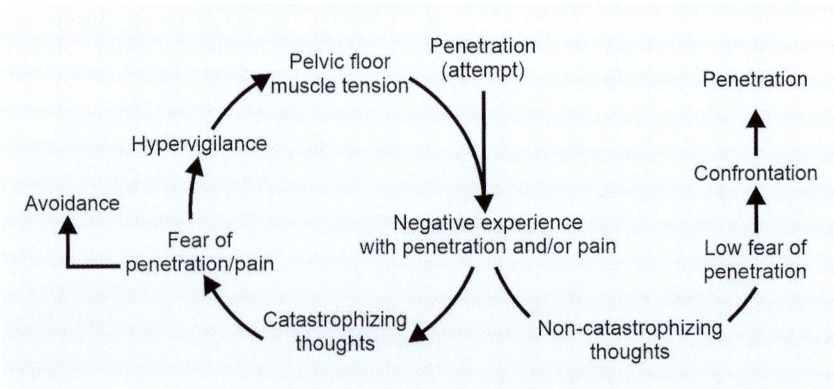

Fig. 1: The fear avoidance model of vaginismus.

The model outline now a negative experience with penetration can lead to catastrophic thinking and resultant fear of treatment, leading to two options:

1. To avoid all activity relating to vaginal penetration.
2. To become hyper-vigilant to stimuli associated with penetration

Hyper-vigilance can lead to exaggerated defensive pelvic muscular contraction, making it difficult to achieve penetration during a subsequent attempt. An inability to achieve penetration might result in more pain and confirm negative experiences associated with penetration. In this way, the experience of vaginismus is then exacerbated and perpetuated in a vicious cycle.

The fear-avoidance model of pain can also be used to conceptualize recovery from vaginismus: with this understanding and acceptance, the result can be reduced fear and ultimately engagement in the activity.

CAUSES AND SYMPTOMS OF VAGINISMUS

There are certain potential causes of vaginismus, and it may be a combination of physical and psychological factors. Understanding the root cause is necessary for finding the right treatment.

Psychological Factors

- *Fear or anxiety:* Negative past experiences such as traumatic sexual experience or abuse can cause fear and anxiety around penetration.
- *Stress:* High level of stress in the relationship or due to personal issue.

Physical Factor

- *Infection or Medical conditions:* Yeast infections, UTIs or pelvic-floor disorders can contribute to vaginal discomfort.
- *Hormonal Changes:* Particularly around menopause and childbirth, can affect the vaginal musculature, leading to dryness and discomfort.
- *Pelvic injury or surgery:* Past surgeries or injuries involving the pelvic area.
- *Cultural or Social influence:* Feeling of spasm or guilt regarding sex can create anxiety.

SYMPTOMS OF VAGINISMUS

- Painful intercourse
- Burning or tingling sensation in the vagina
- Feeling like there is a wall blocking the vagina
- Difficulty inserting a tampon or getting a pelvic exam
- Emotional distress or relationship problem
- Reduced sexual desire or arousalImage

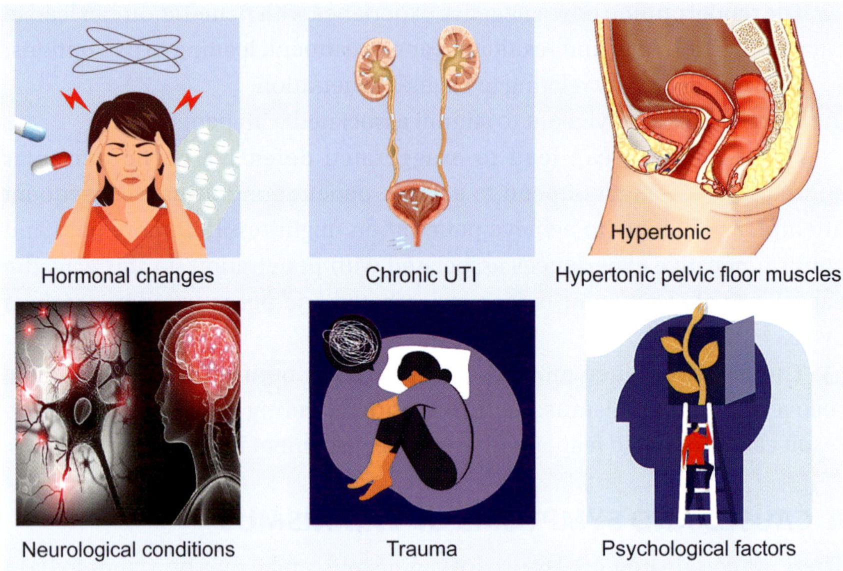

Fig. 2: Causes of vaginismus.

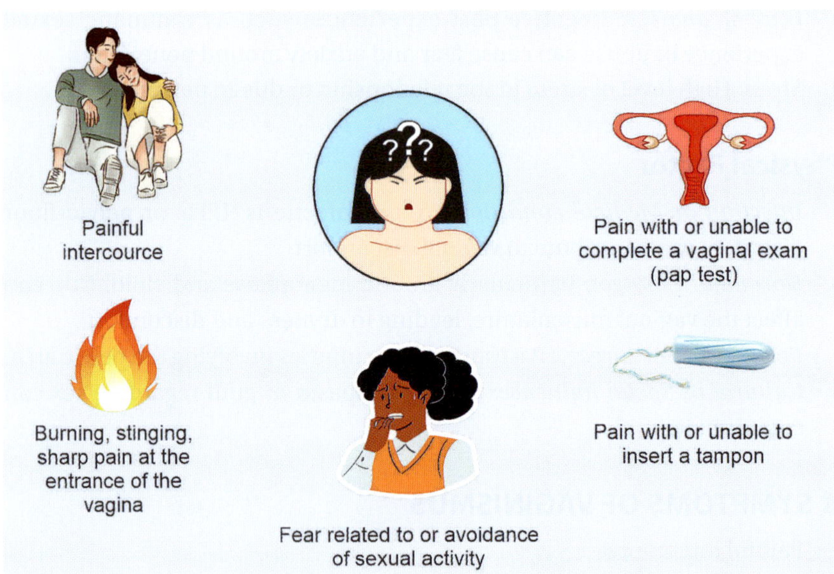

Fig. 3: Symptoms of vaginismus.

DIAGNOSIS

Diagnosing vaginismus can be challenging, particularly as patients often present with concomitant vulval, pelvic floor, and pelvic pain.

In a clinical setting, patients presenting with symptoms suggestive of vaginismus require thorough investigation to make a differential diagnosis and rule out organic comorbidities. Detailed history-taking is important to make an accurate diagnosis of vaginismus, as shown in **Box 1**.

AJGP (Australian Journal of General Practice)

Before diagnosing vaginismus, always rule out secondary causes in women who have difficulty with penetration despite their expressed wish to do so.

BOX 1: Recommended history-taking questions for people with suspected vaginismus.

Pain-specific questions:

- Location of pain - superficial or deep, vulva or vagina
- Onset of pain before, with or after penetration
- Is penetration possible at all?
- Can they insert fingers or a tampon?
- Intensity of pain
- Descriptors of pain - burning, aching, itching
- Chronology of pain if multiple pain sites, what order did they develop?
- Has it been lifelong or acquired?
- What treatments have been trialed?

Medical history:

- Other vaginal symptoms, including discharge, burning and itching
- Comorbid gynecological conditions, including endometriosis, fibroids and other conditions associated with persistent pelvic pain
- Concurrent bladder or bowel symptoms
- History of sexually transmitted diseases
- Any obstetric delivery history of lacerations, episiotomies or other trauma
- History of abdominal or genitourinary surgery or radiation
- History of skin disorders such as eczema, psoriasis or other dermatitis
- Current contraception use
- Current medications: alternative, prescribed, over the counter
- Alcohol and drug use

Psychosocial context:

- Patient's view of the problem and contributing factors
- Has the problem been present in other relationships?
- Willingness of partner(s) to discuss the problem
- History of sexual or physical abuse
- Life stressor contributing factors
- Comorbid depression or anxiety disorders
- Patient goals and what they would consider a satisfactory treatment outcome

People with severe vaginismus often refuse digital vaginal examination. Some patients present with *"pseudo-vaginismus,"* in which they avoid sexual intercourse on purpose.

The criteria for diagnosing vaginismus are based on clinical experience and a review of relevant literature. It consists of *subjective criteria, objective criteria, frequency-duration criteria,* and *exclusion criteria.*

Vaginismus: Proposed diagnostic criteria

1. *Subjective criteria*
    - Persistent and recurrent difficulty or inability to allow vaginal entry of penis, fingers, or any object despite the expressed wish of the female partner due to emotional distress or fear of pain, on anticipation or attempted penetration that is excessive and unreasonable leading to variable avoidance of vaginal penetration.
2. *Objective criteria*
    A. *Clinical criteria*
        - Muscle spasm during vaginal clinical examination-marked tensing and tightening of pelvic floor muscle during attempted vaginal intercourse/penetration
    B. *Laboratory criteria*
        - Increased muscle tone in an EMG study during induction of vaginismus by a vaginal dilator or attempted penetration
3. *Frequency duration criteria*
    - Symptoms persist for 6 months or more, with the inability or difficulty to penetrate during the majority of attempts (>50%)
4. *Exclusion criteria*
    - No secondary cause for pain/difficulty in penetration

TREATMENT

A variety of effective treatments are available to help women overcome vaginismus. These treatments include the use of vaginal dilators, physical therapy with or without biofeedback, sex counseling, psychotherapy, cognitive behavioral therapy (CBT), and the more recent use of *Botox*. Teamwork is the main key to successful treatment, and post-treatment counseling is usually needed.

A *multidisciplinary approach* for vaginismus is recommended, tailored according to the individual's needs.

Physical Therapy

- *Pelvic floor exercise:*
    - Pelvic floor breathing
    - Pelvic floor drops.
    - Kegel exercises.

- *Stretches:*
  - Child's pose
  - Happy Baby pose
  - Deep squats
  - Piriformis stretch

Desensitization Exercise

- *Vaginal dilators:* Using a series of progressively larger vaginal dilators can help to gradually desensitize the pelvic floor muscles and make the patient more comfortable with vaginal penetration.
- *Trigger point release:* A therapist may use gentle pressure to release trigger points in the muscles that are causing pain.

Psychological Behavioral Therapy

- *Cognitive behavioral therapy:* This can help address anxiety, fear, or trauma that may be contributing to the condition by changing negative thought patterns and behaviors.
- *Counseling and psychotherapy:* Counseling is crucial for addressing the psychological dimensions of vaginismus and can help patients process fear or trauma.
- *Couple counseling:* This can be helpful for partners to navigate the condition together and promote understanding, patience, and support.

Medical Treatment

- *Topical Anesthetic cream's:* Creams containing *lidocaine* may be helpful in reducing superficial pain and discomfort during penetration.
- *Medication:* Sometimes, *antidepressant* or *anti-anxiety* drugs may help alleviate associated anxiety or mood disturbances.
- *Botox injection:* In some cases, injection of *botulinum toxin (Botox)* can temporarily paralyze the vaginal muscles, reducing spasms and making penetration easier.

  A dose of *150–400 MIU* was used, and *75% of women achieved satisfactory results* None of the patients given Botox required a second injection, and there were no recurrences or secondary complications during the follow-up period.
- *Surgery:* In rare cases surgery may be considered as the last option. Procedures such as *hymenectomy* or *labiaplasty* may be performed to physically widen the vaginal opening when indicated.

CONCLUSION

Vaginismus is a leading cause of painful sexual intercourse and is characterized by persistent difficulty in allowing vaginal entry of a penis, finger, or object despite the woman's expressed wish to do so. A differential diagnosis of vaginismus can be made through detailed history-taking, genital examination, and a single-digit vaginal examination. Successful treatment of vaginismus is generally *multidisciplinary* and involves a combination of patient education, pelvic floor muscle relaxation, the use of vaginal trainers, and psychological therapy.

TAKE HOME MESSAGES

- It is a real medical condition, not "all in your head" or your fault. It is not a sign of mental weakness, lack of desire, or refusal to engage in intimacy.
- You are not alone. This condition affects many women and is more common than generally perceived.
- Treatment is highly effective. With the right combination of therapies and support, most women can overcome vaginismus and experience comfortable, pain-free penetration.
- A holistic approach is essential. Successful treatment often combines physical and psychological methods.
- Patience and self-compassion are crucial. Recovery is a journey that varies for each individual and takes time. There will be good and bad days, and being kind to yourself is vital for progress.
- Open communication is key. Talking openly with a partner, trusted friend, or healthcare provider can help reduce feelings of isolation, guilt, and embarrassment, and foster a supportive environment for healing.
- Seek professional help. Do not suffer in silence. A healthcare provider, such as a gynecologist or a pelvic floor specialist, can provide an accurate diagnosis and a personalized treatment plan.

KEY POINTS

- We currently lack a full understanding of the etiology of vaginismus, but the *fear-avoidance* model can be helpful in conceptualizing the condition.
- Predisposing factors for vaginismus include both explicit and implicit sociocultural attitudes around sex.
- Validating a person's experience with vaginismus is the *first step* in its management.
- Management should be *multidisciplinary*, including GPs, sexual counsellors, clinical psychologists, physiotherapists, pain specialists, and gynecologists.
- Successful treatment generally involves a *combination* of patient education, pelvic floor muscle relaxation, use of vaginal trainers, and psychological therapy.

SUGGESTED READING

1. Abraham HC. Therapeutic and psychological approach to cases of unconsummated marriage. Br Med J. 1956:837-9.
2. American Psychiatric Association: Diagnostic and Statistical Manual of Mental Disorders, 5th e-Revision (DSM-5-TR). Washington, DC, American Psychiatric Association, 2022. [Internet]
3. Bertolasi L, Frasson E, Cappelletti JY, Vicentini S, Bordignon M, Graziottin A. Botulinum neurotoxin type A injections for vaginismus secondary to vulvar vestibulitis syndrome. Obstet Gynecol. 2009;114(5):1008-1016.

4. Diagnostic and statistical manual of mental disorders, 4th edition. Washington, DC: American Psychiatric Association; 1994. American Psychiatric Association. [Internet]
5. Ghazizadeh S, Nikzad M. Botulinum toxin in the treatment of refractory vaginismus. Obstetrics & Gynecology. 2004;104(5, Part 1):922-5.
6. Har-Toov J, Militscher I, Lessing JB, Abramov L, Chen J. Combined vulvar vestibulitis syndrome with vaginismus: Which to treat first? J Sex Marital Ther. 2001;27(5):521-3. doi:10.1080/713846824. Search PubMed
7. Huguier PC. Dissertation sur quelques points d'anatomie, de physiologie et de pathologie. Medical thesis, Paris, France. 1834. [Google Scholar]
8. Image 1, 2: Created at, ICGL (Indu's Cosmetic Gynecology and Laser Center), Indu Singh, Vaginismus symptoms and causes, image presentation, 2025.
9. Maseroli E, Scavello I, Rastrelli G, Limoncin E, Cipriani S, Corona G, et al. Outcome of medical and psychosexual interventions for vaginismus: A systematic review and meta-analysis. J Sex Med. 2018;15(12):1752-64. doi: 10.1016/j.jsxm.2018.10.003. Search PubMed
10. Pacik PT, Cole JB. When Sex Seems Impossible: Stories of Vaginismus & How You Can Achieve Intimacy: Pewaukee: Odyne publishingPeter Pacik; 2010.1162
11. Pacik PT. Botox treatment for vaginismus. Plastic and Reconstructive Surgery. 2009;124(6):455e-6e.
12. Pacik PT. Vaginismus: review of current concepts and treatment using botox injections, bupivacaine injections, and progres-sive dilation with the patient under anesthesia. Aesthetic Plastic Surgery. 2011;35(6):1160-4.
13. Pacik PT. Vaginismus: review of current concepts and treatment using botox injections, bupivacaine injections, and progressive dilation with the patient under anesthesia. Aesthetic plastic surgery. 2011;35(6):1160-4.
14. Reissing ED, Binik YM, Khalifé S, Cohen D, Amsel R. Vaginal spasm, pain, and behavior: an empirical investigation of the diagnosis of vaginismus. Arch Sex Beh. 2004;33:5-17. doi: 10.1023/B:ASEB.0000007458.32852.c8. [DOI] [PubMed] [Google Scholar]
15. Schnyder U, Schnyder-Lüthi C, Ballinari P, Blaser A. Therapy for vaginismus: In vivo versus in vitro desensitization. Can J Psychiatry 1998;43(9):941-44. doi: 10.1177/070674379804300910. Search PubMed
16. El-Sibai AS, O. Vaginismus: results of treatment with botulin toxin. Journal of Obstetrics & Gynecology. 2000;20(3):300-2.
17. Spector I, Carey M. Incidence and prevalence of the sexual dysfunctions: a critical review of the empirical literature. Arch Sex Behav. 1990;19:389-396. doi: 10.1007/BF01541933. [DOI] [PubMed] [Google Scholar]
18. ter Kuile MM, Reissing E. Lifelong vaginismus. In: Binik YM, Hall KSK, editors. Principles and practice of sex therapy,. 5th edition. New York: The Guildford Press, 2014. Search PubMed
19. Vlaeyen JWS, Linton SJ. Fear-avoidance and its consequences in chronic musculoskeletal pain: A state of the art. Pain 2000;85(3):317-32. doi: 10.1016/S0304-3959(99)00242-0. Search PubMed

6

CHAPTER

Menopause and Sexuality

Swapnita Hota

INTRODUCTION

Menopause is a natural physiological event signifying the end of a woman's reproductive phase, usually between 45–55 years of age, caused by the decline in ovarian hormone production. This transition is often accompanied by vasomotor, psychological, and sexual symptoms that may affect quality of life.

The consequent decline in estrogen and androgen levels leads to urogenital atrophy, collectively termed Genitourinary Syndrome of Menopause (GSM).

Sexuality during menopause is shaped by hormonal changes, emotional well-being, and partner relationships. Declining estrogen and androgen levels can lead to vaginal dryness, dyspareunia, and reduced libido, while psychological and cultural factors further influence sexual satisfaction. Addressing these changes through counseling, lifestyle modification, and individualized therapy is essential for maintaining sexual health and overall well-being. **Table 1** describes the physiological changes in menopause.

Psychosocial and Relationship Factors

- *Body image concerns:* Weight gain, skin changes, aging signs reduce self-confidence.
- *Partner's sexual health:* Erectile dysfunction or chronic illness of any of partner (e.g., Diabetes, hypertension, chronic heart diseases, osteoarthritis, neurological disease, *obesity*, vascular diseases) can compound sexual difficulties.
- *Cultural silence:* In many societies, discussing sexual issues is taboo, leading to neglect.
- *Emotional factors:* Fear of rejection, anxiety, depression or past-trauma may affect sexual behavior. **Table 2** illustrates the common sexual issues that happen in menopausal women.

CLINICAL EVALUATION

- *History:* Focusing 6-key components desire, arousal, lubrication, orgasm, satisfaction, pain.
- *Quantitative assessment tools:* Female sexual function index, menopause specific quality of life questionnaire (FSFI, MENQOL) help in baseline evaluation and monitoring response to therapy.

TABLE 1: Physiological changes in menopause affecting sexuality.

Change	*Description*	*Effect on sexuality*
Decline in estrogen	• Leads to decreased vascularity thinning of vaginal mucosa, decreased lactobacilli changing vaginal flora leading to recurrent vaginal infections • Decreased vaginal elasticity due to decreased collagen and elastin • Denervation	Vaginal dryness, dyspareunia, decreased sexual satisfaction
• Decline in progesterone • Decline in testosterone	• Altered neuro-endocrine regulation • Contributes to decreased libido and energy levels	• Hypoactive sexual desire, arousal difficulties • Reduced sexual desire, fatigue
Decline in pelvic muscle tone, pelvic organ prolapse	Weakens orgasmic response	Reduced satisfaction
Vasomotor symptoms	Hot flashes, night sweats	Sleep disturbance, fatigue
Mood changes	Anxiety, depression	Lower self-image, reduced intimacy

TABLE 2: Common sexual dysfunctions in menopausal women.

Dysfunction	*Description*	*Prevalence*	*Contributing factors*
Hypoactive sexual desire disorder	Persistent lack of desire for sexual activity	30–50%	Hormonal decline, stress
Arousal disorder	Difficulty in attaining or maintaining arousal	20–30%	Vaginal dryness, anxiety
Orgasmic disorder	Delay or absence of orgasm	15–25%	Pelvic muscle weakness
Dyspareunia	Painful intercourse	20–40%	GSM
Sexual aversion disorder	Avoidance due to pain or negative experiences	10–15%	Psychological distress

- *Physical examination:* Genital health-vulvovaginal atrophy, loss of rugosities, elasticity, lesion or tenderness.
- *Laboratory test:* Serum estradiol, progesterone, total/free testosterone, SHBG, LH/FSH, TSH, metabolic profile.

MANAGEMENT APPROACH

Counseling and Education

- Normalize discussion regarding sexual health during menopause.
- Encourage partner participation to enhance communication and emotional intimacy.
- Emphasize women that sexual activity remains safe and beneficial in midlife and beyond.

Lifestyle Modifications

- *BE ACTIVE:* Regular walking/aerobics; yoga (Squat/Malasana, Balasana, Viparita Virasana, Bridge pose) breathing exercises, pelvic floor strengthening exercises (Kegels), strength training, meditation.
- Balanced diet rich in phytoestrogens and omega-3 fatty acids.
- Adequate sleep and stress management.
- *Avoid alcohol and other drugs:* slower body response.
- *Avoid smoking:* reduces blood flow to vagina and lowers estrogen effects.
- *Pelvic floor exercises:* increased blood flow to vagina and strengthens pelvic muscles.

Therapeutic options for menopausal sexual symptoms are summarized in **Table 3**.

Psychosexual Therapy

- Cognitive behavioral therapy.
- Couple therapy for intimacy
    - *Have sex more often:* it can increase blood flow to your vagina and help keep tissues healthy.
    - *Allow time to become aroused (Foreplay):* Moisture from being aroused protects tissues and makes sex more comfortable.

Emerging Treatments

BHRT: Bioidentical hormone replacement therapy involves use of hormone chemically identical to those naturally produced in human body, derived from plant sources, e.g., soy and yam and modified to match human hormones.

FEMININE ESTHETICS AND REJUVENATION

Nonsurgical and Regenerative Therapies

- PRP (Platelet-Rich Plasma)/PRF (Platelet rich fibrin): Autologous growth factors promote angiogenesis and tissue rejuvenation. Used as orgasmic shots "O-shot" "G-shot" for clitoral and vaginal sensitivity and rejuvenation, suburethral shots for urinary incontinence.

TABLE 3: Vaginal and hormonal therapies in menopause (HRT).

Category	*Drugs*	*Dose*	*Indications and use*	*Side effects*	*Safety and monitoring*
Estrogen therapy	Conjugated equine estrogen (CEE), 17-β Estradiol, Estradiol patch/gel, Vaginal estrogen cream/ring	*Oral:* CEE 0.3–0.625 mg/day; Estradiol 0.5–2 mg/day, *Patch:* 25–100 µg/day (3–4 days), Vaginal gel 0.5–1 g daily × 2 weeks, then 2×/week, 6–12 months	Vasomotor symptoms, vaginal dryness, no uterus	Breast tenderness, bloating headache	C/I in breast endometrial ca, VTE, liver disease Transdermal route safer. Monitor 6–12 months
Combined (E+P)	Estradiol + micronized progesterone, CEE + MPA	Estradiol 1 mg + MP100 mg daily, sequential CEE0.625 mg CEE + MPA 0.625mg CEE/5mg MPA	Women with intact uterus-prevent endometrial hyperplasia, vasomotor symptoms	Irregular bleeding, breast tenderness, bloating	Breast ca risk ↑ with MPA >5 years Safer with micronized progesterone, avoid in suspected ca
Progesterone only	Micronized progesterone, MPA, LNG-IUS	MP 100/200 mg, MPA 2.5–10 mg/day for 12–14 days/cycle	Where estrogen C/I	Breast tenderness, irregular bleeding	Protective breast/endometrium, LNG-IUS safer
Testosterone	Transdermal gel/patch	300 mcg/day topical	Hypoactive sexual desire disorder (HSDD)	Acne, hirsutism, oily skin	Avoid in androgen sensitive ca, safe short term <2 years
Local vaginal therapies	Vaginal estrogen (cream/tab/ring), progesterone vaginal suppositories	Estradiol 0.01% cream	Genitourinary syndrome of menopause (GSM)	Local irritation	Safe
SERMs	Ospemifene/raloxifene	60 mg/day	Vaginal atrophy/dyspareunia, osteoporosis prevention	Hot flashes, leg cramps	Avoid in history of of VTE
Tibolone	Livial	2.5 mg/day	Vasomotor symptom, low libido	Weight gain, spotting	C/I breast ca, increased stroke risk
Non-hormonal lubricants		Water-based gels (Lubic gel)	Reduces dyspareunia		Avoid irritants (bubble bath, soaps)

- Stem Cell Therapy (Adipose-derived/Mesenchymal): Regenerates collagen and enhances tissue trophism for GSM and vulvar dystrophy, used as filler.

Energy-based Devices

CO_2 Laser (Fractional/Microablative) 10,600 nm. Causes controlled micro-thermal injury → collagen remodeling and neovascularization Uses-Vaginal laxity, GSM (genitourinary syndrome of menopause), stress urinary incontinence, vulvar dystrophy.

Er:YAG Laser (Erbium:Yttrium-Aluminum-Garnet) 2940 nm. Non-ablative, superficial heating; stimulates fibroblast activity uses-Vaginal dryness, mild prolapse, vaginal tightening, atrophic vaginitis.

Nd:YAG Laser1064 nm Deeper tissue penetration; heating of collagen fibers and connective tissue Combined use with Er:YAG for tightening and vulvar rejuvenation (CO_2/Er:YAG),whitening and lightens vulvar pigmentation. Stimulation of collagen, tightening of vaginal mucosa, improves lubrication, dyspareunia, and orgasmic response.

Radiofrequency (RF) Therapy: Controlled thermal effect increases collagen remodeling. Safe, minimal downtime; enhances vaginal tone. Uses-GSM, SUI, vulvar dystrophy, vaginal tightening.

HIFU (High intensity focused ultrasound waves): Noninvasive energy to deeper tissue layers for vaginal tightening, improves sexual function in menopausal women with laxity and atrophy.

Genital Peels/Chemical Peels

Improve pigmentation, texture and tone of vulvar and perineal skin by exfoliation of epidermis. Uses: boost self-confidence.

Surgical Procedure

- Labiaplasty (Labia minora reduction) for elongated or asymmetric labia causing discomfort or self-consciousness. Enhances sexual confidence, genital esthetics
- *Clitoral Hood Reduction:* Improves clitoral exposure and sexual stimulation often combined with labiaplasty.
- Vaginoplasty (Perineal tightening) Tightens vaginal canal; improves frictional sensation, can be surgical or non-surgical (laser/RF) or combined.
- *Fat Grafting/Filler Injections:* Restores vulvar volume, corrects labial atrophy, Hyaluronic acid or autologous fat (nano fat)commonly used
- *Monsplasty:* Addresses ptosis. Improves aesthetic appeal, self-esteem.

KEY POINTS

- Menopause causes biological and emotional transitions influencing sexuality.
- Hormonal decline leads to vaginal dryness, reduced libido, and dyspareunia.
- Psychological and partner related factors significantly modulate sexual well-being.
- Holistic management, patient-centered approach combining counseling, lifestyle modification and medical therapy is effective.
- Local estrogen therapy remains first-line for genitourinary syndrome of menopause.
- Open communication with partner and provider is key.
- Menopause should be seen as a phase of renewal and empowerment not decline.

SUGGESTED READING

1. American College of Obstetricians and Gynecologists. Elective female genital cosmetic surgery. Committee Opinion No. 795. Obstet Gynecol. 2020;135(1):e36-42.
2. Baber RJ, Panay N, Fenton A; IMS Writing Group. 2016 IMS recommendations on women's midlife health and menopause hormone therapy. Climacteric. 2016;19(2):109-50.
3. Davis SR, Baber R, Panay N, Bitzer J, Cerdas Perez S, Islam RM, et al. Global consensus position statement on the use of testosterone therapy for women. Climacteric. 2019;22(5):429-34.
4. Dennerstein L. Sexuality and the menopause. J Br Menopause Soc. 2005;11(1):22-6.
5. Hilditch JR, Lewis J, Peter A, van Maris B, Ross A, Franssen E, et al. A menopause-specific quality of life questionnaire: development and psychometric properties. Maturitas. 1996;24(3):161-75.
6. International Society of Cosmetic Gynecology (ISCG). Guidelines 2021: functional and aesthetic energy-based devices. New Jersey, USA: ISCG Guidelines; 2021.
7. Kingsberg SA. Hormones and sexual function in postmenopausal women. Obstet Gynecol Clin North Am. 2015;42(4):593-606.
8. Kingsberg SA. The role of androgens in female sexual function. J Sex Med. 2014;11(6):1594-607.
9. Nappi RE. Female sexual dysfunction during menopause. Climacteric. 2019;22(3):233-40.
10. North American Menopause Society. Nonhormonal management of menopause-associated vasomotor symptoms: position statement. Menopause. 2023;30(6):573-90.
11. North American Menopause Society. The 2022 hormone therapy position statement of the North American Menopause Society. Menopause. 2022;29(7):767-94.
12. Rosen R, Brown C, Heiman J, Leiblum S, Meston C, Shabsigh R, et al. The Female Sexual Function Index (FSFI): a multidimensional self-report instrument for the assessment of female sexual function. J Sex Marital Ther. 2000;26(2):191-208.
13. Shifren JL. The menopause transition and sexual function. Menopause. 2022;29(8):912-20.

7 CHAPTER

Sex in Pregnancy

Vani Puri

INTRODUCTION

Pregnancy brings significant physical, psychological, and hormonal changes, along with shifts in overall quality of life and sexual relationships. During this time, many women experience deeper emotional bonding, increased intimacy, and a heightened need for physical closeness, all of which are intertwined with sexual expression and pleasure.

Research indicates that women often lack structured or accurate information about sexual activity during pregnancy, which can contribute to unnecessary worries. Persistent myths—such as the belief that intercourse can harm the fetus or trigger preterm labor or miscarriage—remain powerful sources of fear and may lead couples to avoid sexual contact during pregnancy.

Sexual behavior in pregnancy is also shaped by a range of influences, including sociocultural norms, demographic background, religious beliefs, educational level, length of the relationship, financial stability, gestational age, and whether the pregnancy was planned. In this context, sexuality is understood as the combination of identity, emotions, and behaviors related to sexual expression.

PREGNANCY: A REMARKABLE JOURNEY FILLED WITH DEMANDS

How a pregnant couple feels, their thoughts, acceptance towards pregnancy, and attitude towards sexuality during pregnancy depends upon how the partners decided to conceive (planned/unplanned). A well-planned conception increases enjoyment and consequently sexuality during this time.

It is very common for a pregnant woman to experience pregnancy as a loss of self-identity and to feel that her body does not belong to her, while pregnancy is a celebration for the rest of the family. Partner support and attention can strongly impact the woman's feelings during pregnancy. However, even if pregnancy was desired by both, it is normal to have ambivalent feelings.

Pregnancy can be a demanding phase not only for the expectant mother but also for her partner. Some may struggle with doubts about their career, future responsibilities, and readiness for parenthood. As the woman's focus gradually shifts from being a partner to preparing for motherhood, the dynamics of the relationship may naturally change. This makes open communication essential. Talking honestly about emotions, fears, and expectations during pregnancy helps prevent misunderstandings from growing into bigger issues. When these emotional concerns are ignored, they can gradually strain the couple's bond and negatively influence their intimacy and overall relationship wellbeing.

PHYSIOLOGICAL AND PSYCHOLOGICAL CHANGES AFFECTING SEXUALITY

Physiological Changes

During the first trimester, common symptoms such as missed periods, nausea, and persistent tiredness are normal but often uncomfortable. These physical changes can reduce sexual desire and make arousal more difficult.

In the second trimester, the enlargement and tenderness of the breasts may cause discomfort for some women, while others may feel more feminine and confident. Increased blood flow to the pelvic region heightens genital sensitivity, which can make orgasms easier to achieve and may enhance sexual desire.

By the third trimester, many women experience a sense of heaviness, breathlessness, fatigue, and disturbed sleep due to frequent urination. The growing uterus can also create a feeling of awkwardness or reduced mobility, which may influence body image and self-confidence.

Psychological Changes

During pregnancy, a woman typically moves through three psychological stages of acceptance, and these shifting emotional focuses can significantly influence her sexual interest. In the first trimester, her attention is primarily directed inward as she processes how pregnancy will alter her life.

In the second trimester, her focus gradually shifts toward the developing baby, especially as she begins to feel fetal movements. This stage often brings stronger protective instincts and a deeper emotional connection with the unborn child.

By the third trimester, the approaching birth becomes central in her mind. This awareness may trigger anxiety related to her own safety and that of the baby. Concerns about body image and the discomfort caused by physical changes are also common during this period.

Social Changes

A woman's acceptance of pregnancy is strongly influenced by cultural beliefs, the way pregnancy is represented in the media, and the reactions of people close to her—especially her partner. Because she experiences visible and physical changes, the reality of becoming a parent feels more immediate to her than to her partner. For many partners, the recognition that their roles will soon shift often develops later. This difference in timing can create strain in the relationship, making it helpful for couples to openly discuss and understand this "adjustment gap" in embracing future parenthood.

Couvade syndrome: Although partners of pregnant women typically do not undergo physical changes, some may experience psychosomatic symptoms that mirror the woman's fatigue, nausea, or general discomfort. Research suggests that this syndrome may be associated with hormonal shifts in the male partner, including reduced levels of cortisol and testosterone, which can in turn lower sexual desire. Couvade syndrome is reported more frequently in first-time pregnancies and in pregnancies that were not planned.

SEXUALITY IN PREGNANCY: DIVERSITY OF NORMALCY

In a healthy, uncomplicated pregnancy, couples can safely continue sexual activity throughout the entire term. However, their level of desire often shifts as pregnancy progresses. Several studies note a reduction in sexual activity during these nine months, while a few report that some couples maintain regular intercourse right up to childbirth. More commonly, sexual frequency declines—sometimes by as much as 50%. Some partners even stop sexual activity immediately after learning about the pregnancy.

Typically, there is a mild decrease in intercourse during the first trimester, a slight rise in the second trimester, and a marked decline in the third trimester. Sexual desire, arousal, and the ability to reach orgasm during pregnancy vary greatly among women. These changes differ not only from one woman to another but also from one pregnancy to the next, and even across different trimesters. The quality of the couple's relationship and their overall satisfaction with the partnership play a major role in shaping these experiences.

COUNSELING SEXUALITY TO PREGNANT COUPLES: OVERCOMING THE TABOO

Many healthcare professionals hesitate to discuss sexual matters with pregnant couples, often explaining that they wish to respect the couple's privacy. However, couples frequently expect clinicians to initiate this conversation. Sexuality during pregnancy is sometimes obscured by using vague terms like *intimacy* when the intended meaning is sexual activity. Miscommunication can also arise when the word *sex* is used to refer only to penetration.

Ideally, discussions about sexual health in pregnancy should begin during pre-pregnancy counseling or early in the first trimester. Both partners should be included in conversations about sexuality, with individual sessions offered if needed.

Some sexual concerns can be resolved quickly. For instance, guidance on alternative sexual positions can reduce abdominal pressure in late pregnancy and ease anxiety in low-risk couples. Many women find positions such as woman-on-top, side-lying, or rear-entry more comfortable as the uterus enlarges. Providing clear information about the safety of the baby during intercourse is also important. Discussing non-coital forms of sexual expression that both partners find acceptable can help couples manage differences in desire.

Some couples may also need support in managing tension caused by unmet sexual needs. Non-penetrative sexual activities can be especially useful during the third trimester and early postpartum period. Exploring sensual touch, outercourse, and new forms of intimacy may feel unfamiliar but can effectively reduce frustration. This process is often referred to as *renegotiating intimacy.*

Pregnant women often receive confusing or inaccurate advice from various sources. Healthcare providers should proactively address sexuality to dispel myths, challenge cultural misconceptions, and reduce unnecessary fears or anxieties. These discussions must always be conducted with empathy, respect, and cultural awareness.

CONCLUSION

Sexual behavior during pregnancy is shaped by a combination of hormonal, emotional, and social influences, highlighting the biopsychosocial nature of sexuality. These interacting factors often create a sexual experience that differs significantly from pre-pregnancy life. A woman's level of sexual desire may be lower or higher than her partner's, and she may struggle with changes in her body image. Similarly, her partner may find it challenging to adjust to the transition from seeing his partner as a lover to seeing her as a mother.

Partners may also experience mixed emotions about the pregnancy, even when they strongly desire a child. Some may feel excluded, as the pregnant woman naturally becomes the focus of attention for family, friends, and healthcare providers. Because each couple's situation is unique, there is no universal guideline for advising all pregnant women and their partners about sexual activity. However, supporting their sexual wellbeing remains an important component of overall health.

This underscores the need for healthcare professionals—particularly obstetricians and midwives—to take a more active role in educating and guiding couples about sexual health during pregnancy. Providing clear, empathetic, and evidence-based information can help couples navigate this period with confidence and maintain a healthy intimate relationship.

KEY POINTS

- Pregnancy reshapes intimacy through physical, psychological, and hormonal changes.
- Myths about sex harming the fetus often cause fear and avoidance.
- Planned pregnancies usually enhance sexual satisfaction and bonding.
- Open communication prevents misunderstandings and strengthens relationships.
- First trimester symptoms often reduce sexual desire.
- Second trimester sensitivity can boost arousal and confidence.
- Third trimester discomfort and body image concerns lower sexual activity.
- Partners may experience Couvade Syndrome, mirroring pregnancy symptoms.
- Sexual activity is safe in uncomplicated pregnancies though frequency declines.
- Counselling dispels myths, suggests positions, and promotes nonpenetrative intimacy.

SUGGESTED READING

1. Abdool Z, Thakar R, Sultan AH. Sexual function during pregnancy and postpartum. Nat Rev Urol. 2020;17(5):285-302.
2. ACOG Committee Opinion No. 808: Sexual activity during uncomplicated pregnancy. Obstet Gynecol. 2020;135(5):e215-20.
3. Brennan PA, Hancock P. Couvade syndrome: psychosomatic and hormonal changes in expectant fathers. J Psychosom Obstet Gynaecol. 2021;42(4):289-96.
4. Fagundes CP, Diamond LM. Cultural and relational influences on sexuality during pregnancy. Arch Sex Behav. 2021;50(3):1125-38.
5. Fernández-Carrasco FJ, Batugg-Chaves C, Ruger-Navarrete A, Riesco-González FJ, Palomo-Gómez R, Gómez-Salgado J, et al. Influence of pregnancy on sexual desire in pregnant women and their partners: a systematic review. Public Health Rev. 2023;44:1606308.
6. Gutiérrez-Martínez O, Sánchez-Sánchez A. Psychological adaptation stages in pregnancy and their impact on sexuality. Women Birth. 2022;35(6):e556-63.
7. Rezaei N, Azadi A, Sayehmiri K. Comfortable sexual positions in late pregnancy: a clinical review. BMC Pregnancy Childbirth. 2021;21(1):712.
8. Rosen NO, Muise A. Maintaining intimacy during pregnancy: non-penetrative sexual strategies and couple adjustment. J Sex Res. 2024;61(2):245-57.
9. Vannier SA, Rosen NO. The role of pregnancy planning in sexual satisfaction among expectant couples. J Sex Med. 2022;19(4):613-21.
10. Vázquez-Lara JM, Palomo-Gómez R, Díaz LR. Patterns of sexual activity across pregnancy: a longitudinal study. Int J Gynaecol Obstet. 2023;162(2):456-62.

8 CHAPTER

Media Influence on Sexual Health

Tripti Sharan

DEFINITION OF SEXUAL HEALTH

- Sexual health is a state of physical, emotional, mental and social well-being, not merely the absence of disease or dysfunction.
- It requires a positive and respectful approach to sexuality and relationships.
- Every individual should be able to experience pleasurable and safe sexual experiences free from coercion and violence.

MEDIA AND SEXUAL HEALTH

- Media is a central influence shaping society's view of sexuality.
- Youth spend around 6–7 hours daily on TV, OTT, music and social media.
- The mix of entertainment and education often blurs the boundary between knowledge and misinformation.
- Unfiltered exposure affects attitudes toward gender, relationships and sexual behavior.

SEXUAL CONTENT IN MEDIA

- Nearly two-thirds of TV/OTT shows contain sexual content.
- Around 20–50% of music videos show sexual imagery.
- For every 25 scenes of sexual behavior, only one shows protective practice like contraception or consent.
- Lack of realistic outcomes (such as STIs, pregnancy, emotional impact) creates false perceptions especially amongst adolescents.
- Leads to normalization of risky sexual behavior among viewers.

VULNERABLE POPULATIONS

- Adolescents report media as their main source of sexual information, while only ≈11% learn from parents.
- Girls are exposed to relationship-based themes; boys to dominance and fantasy-driven content.
- Cultural and religious contexts shape how messages are interpreted.
- Influences attitudes on gender roles and intimacy.

INTERPRETATION AND BEHAVIOR

- Media messages are interpreted differently by age, gender and culture.
- *Frequent exposure is linked with:*
  - Early sexual initiation
  - Risk-taking behavior and normalization of risky behavior
  - Poor understanding of consent and boundaries
  - Body objectification and unrealistic expectations
- Repeated exposure desensitizes youth to intimacy and real emotional connections.

PSYCHOLOGICAL AND SOCIAL EFFECTS

- Excess sexualized content can cause anxiety, body image issues and low self-esteem.
- Problematic porn use linked to erectile dysfunction and low satisfaction.
- Sexting and cyberbullying exposes youth to emotional trauma and legal complications.
- Creates distorted notions of love and relationships.

CHILD SEXUAL ABUSE AND GROOMING

- CSA involves using a child in sexual activity that they cannot understand or consent to.
- Sexual grooming is a gradual process involving trust-building before exploitation.
- *Common stages include:*
  1. Targeting the child
  2. Gaining trust
  3. Meeting emotional needs
  4. Isolating the child
  5. Sexualizing the relationship
  6. Maintaining control
- Occurs online or offline, across all genders and ages.

POSITIVE IMPACT OF MEDIA

- When used responsibly, media can promote sexual health awareness and inclusivity.
- Provides access to accurate information on STIs, contraception and consent.
- Breaks social taboos and normalizes open discussion.
- Encourages support for marginalized groups and reduces stigma.

ROLE OF PROFESSIONALS

- Guide adolescents to develop media literacy.

- Encourage communication between youth and parents.
- Promote informed decision-making and realistic understanding of relationships and sexuality.
- Advocate responsible media portrayal of sexuality and consent.

WAYS TO USE MEDIA POSITIVELY

- Encourage blogging
- Use social media for live lectures
- Create interest based Facebook groups
- Use Pinterest boards
- Use You tube for presentations
- Use Twitter for concise discussion and debates
- Use social media pages to postinformation and spread awareness on relevant issues
- Be a part of Quora discussions
- Build professional connections
- Find teaching resources on social media

SEXUALITY EDUCATION

- Sexuality education extends beyond biology to include emotional intelligence, gender identity, consent, intimacy, and body image.
- It equips adolescents with scientific, age-appropriate information, empowering them to make informed choices.
- Myths such as "sex education encourages early sex" are unfounded.
- Research confirms that comprehensive sexuality education delays sexual initiation and reduces unprotected sexual activity and STIs.

RESPONSIBLE SEXUAL BEHAVIOR (ABCD MODEL)

A - Abstinence
B - Be Faithful
C - Condom/Contraceptives
D - Disease Alert and Testing

- Maintain a balance between fantasy and reality.
- Avoid addiction, ensure consent, and stay legally aware.
- Child pornography is punishable by law.
  Ethical responsibility is central to healthy sexuality.

RECOMMENDATIONS

- *Adopt a multilevel approach:*
  - *Individual:* Counselling and awareness
  - *Institutional:* Media literacy programs in schools
  - *Governmental:* Regulation, warning labels, and awareness campaigns

- Train clinicians and educators to handle sexuality-related issues sensitively.
- Promote digital hygiene and healthy media habits.

CONCLUSION

- Media is a powerful educator and influencer.
- Its effects depend on content, audience, and interpretation.
- Through proactive education, regulation and awareness, it can become a constructive force promoting healthy sexuality, equality and safety.

KEY POINTS

- Sexual health covers physical, emotional and social well-being.
- Media strongly influences sexual perceptions and behavior.
- Overexposure may lead to risky sexual behavior and body image issues.
- Responsible media and sexuality education empower safer choices.
- Professionals should foster media literacy and awareness.
- Regulation and parental guidance are vital to balance fantasy and reality.

SUGGESTED READING

1. Brown JD, Greenberg BS, Buerkel-Rothfuss NL. Mass media, sex, and sexuality. Adolesc Med. 1993;4(pt 1):511-52. [PubMed] [Google Scholar]
2. Brown JD. Mass Media Influences on Sexuality. J Adolesc Health. 2002;39(1):42-5.
3. Bull SS, Levine DK, Black SR, Schmiege SJ, Santelli J. Social media–Delivered sexual health intervention. American Journal of Preventive Medicine. 2012;43:467-474. doi: 10.1016/j.amepre.2012.07.022. [DOI] [PMC free article] [PubMed] [Google Scholar]
4. Finkelhor D. Child Sexual Abuse: New Theory and Research. New York: Free Press; 1984.
5. Kinsler JJ, Glik D, de Castro Buffington S, Malan H, Nadjat-Haiem C, Wainwright N, et al. A Content Analysis of How Sexual Behavior and Reproductive Health are Being Portrayed on Primetime Television Shows Being Watched by Teens and Young Adults. Health Commun. 2019;34(6):644-51.
6. Kirby DB, Laris BA, Rolleri LA. Impact of Comprehensive Sex Education on Adolescent Sexual Behavior. J Adolesc Health. 2007;40(3):206-17.
7. Kunkel D, Cope KM, Maynard-Farinola WJ, et al. Sex on TV: content and context. Menlo Park (CA): Kaiser Family Foundation; 1999.
8. Park BY, Wilson G, Berger J, Christman M, Reina B, Bishop F, et al. Is Internet Pornography Causing Sexual Dysfunction? J Sex Med. 2016;13(6):918-31.
9. UNESCO. International Technical Guidance on Sexuality Education. Paris: UNESCO: 2018.
10. World Health Organization. Defining sexual health. Geneva: WHO; 2006.

9 CHAPTER

Erectile Dysfunction

Aatmik Jain

DEFINITION

International Consultation on Sexual Dysfunctions defines *erectile dysfunction* as "the persistent inability to attain and maintain an erection sufficient to permit satisfactory sexual performance".

Minimum duration: 3 months (Safie Kirana, et al.).

PHYSIOLOGY OF NORMAL ERECTION

The parasympathetic pathway through the pelvic splanchnic nerve plexuses and pudendal nerve causes the penis cavernosal tissue to release nitric oxide (NO).

NO, with the help of cyclic guanosine monophosphate, reduces intracellular calcium, and the cavernosal smooth muscle relaxes.

Blood rushes into cavernosal tissues and obstructs venous outflow; thus, erection is maintained as veins are compressed against the tunica albuginea.

The rhythmic contraction of the cavernosal smooth muscle is done by adrenergic receptor activation, which causes a decrease in arterial size and induces venous outflow, thus causing detumescence.

PATHOPHYSIOLOGY

Psychological Status of Men with Erectile Dysfunction

Self-confidence of men with ED shatters, resulting in a decline in their ability to achieve an erection.

Men with severe organic ED also have a psychological component. The psychological characteristics of men with severe ED are poorer than those with mild ED.

It has been seen in clinics that some men diagnosed with mild or nonorganic ED find it more distressing and report it as "severe". On the other hand, if they receive treatment earlier for necessary sexual acts, their confidence improves drastically.

Depression and ED

Several studies have shown that patients with depression have 39% higher risk of ED, and in patients with ED risk of depression increases by 192%, than those without both these conditions.

The behavioral model to explain this relationship states that depressive patients have negative thoughts and poor confidence, resulting in performance anxiety and further reduction of erection quality.

The biological model states that depression affects the hypothalamic-pituitary-adrenocortical (HPA) axis, causing increased catecholamine secretion and, in turn, poor cavernosal muscle relaxation.

At last, many antidepressant drugs have negative effects on erectile function.

Metabolic Syndrome and ED

The proinflammatory state of Metabolic syndromes leads to endothelial dysfunction and reduces the availability of nitric oxide.

In ED, it is seen that there are reduced vascular NO and cellular antioxidants, but increased superoxide radicals.

These superoxide radicals, along with oxidized LDL, are responsible for impairment of endothelial NO and thus hampering endothelial relaxation and developing ED.

Hypercholesterolemia is characterized by impaired cavernous smooth muscle relaxation in various vascular beds, causing ED.

Obesity and ED

Enzyme aromatase is increased in visceral fat, which is responsible for the conversion of testosterone to estrogen and the synthesis of leptin protein. This protein is inversely associated with testosterone levels.

Diabetes and Erectile Dysfunction

The proposed mechanisms behind the causality of ED due to diabetes include psychogenic factors, hyperglycemia, impaired nitric oxide synthesis, cGMP and RhoA/Rho-kinase pathway disruption, neuropathic damage, and downregulation of growth factors and neurotransmitters' gene expression affecting neuronal and inducible nitric oxide synthase.

Testosterone and ED

There is a reduction seen in serum testosterone levels by the age of 40.

Studies in castrated men showed complete or partial ED, low libido, poor orgasms, and spontaneous and nocturnal erections due to low serum testosterone.

The main mechanism is a reduction in cavernous vasodilation in men due to low testosterone levels.

CAD and ED

According to the "artery size" hypothesis, larger vessels are affected later than smaller ones by the same degree of atherosclerotic plaque development.

Therefore, when the coronary circulation is impacted, the penile circulation has already experienced more damage.

ED should appear before CAD, and CAD patients should have frequent ED.

DIAGNOSTIC ASSESSMENT

Initial Assessment of a Patient with ED

Medical History

For assessing psychogenic ED, we can use the Leiden Impotence Screening Test (LIST).

For assessing organic ED, one should focus on past medical history, including the patient's lifestyle habits like diet, smoking, alcohol, drug abuse, and prescribed medicines.

Sexual History

For this purpose, we can use questionnaires International Index of Erectile Function (IIEF), Erectile Dysfunction Inventory of Treatment Satisfaction (EDITS), Brief Male Sexual Function Inventory and sexological mini-anamnesis.

Physical Examination

Focused physical examination is a must, which includes BMI, body weight, body habitus, cardiovascular and neurological.

Genital examination should include penile, testicular and rectal examination to rule out micropenis, phimosis, Peyronie's disease, prostate diseases, etc.

Diagnostic Tests

Initial assessment with: Early morning samples (between 8 and 10 AM) of blood glucose, total testosterone, TSH and prolactin, lipid profile.

Further evaluation: Free testosterone, sex hormone binding globulin, thyroid profile, FSH and LH.

Vascular Evaluation

1. *Office Sildenafil test*: Oral Sildenafil citrate (50 mg or 100mg) is given to the patient and can be combined with genital stimulation and/or visual erotic stimulation (VES). Erection quality is seen after 1 hour.
2. *Penile pharmacologic duplex ultrasound (PPDU):* A vasoactive drug (usually 10–20 mg prostaglandin E1) is injected into the cavernosal tissue of the penis for the assessment of arterial insufficiency and veno-occlusive functions. Peak systolic velocity (PSV), End diastolic flow velocity (EDV)

and resistance index (RI) are seen. The diagnosis is considered when PSV >30 cm/s and EDV >3–5 cm/sec or RI <0.9, concluding a veno-occlusive disease and arteriogenic insufficiency when PSV <25–30 cm/s.

3. *Penile arteriography:* Internal pudendal arteries and their outflow tracts are seen. Mainly used in young men with a history of pelvic/perineal trauma.
4. *Nocturnal Penile Tumescence and Rigidity:* Night-time and early morning erections are normal physiological events and are associated with REM sleep.
   Method: Patient is asked to sleep in a quiet room. 2 circular strain gauges are applied to the tip and base of the penis. An overnight recording of >70% rigidity, 3–4 erections lasting for >10 minutes are considered normal values.
5. Dynamic Infusion Cavernosometry/Cavernosography:
   Method: Use a 19-G butterfly needle in each corpus cavernosa and inject 20 mg prostaglandin E1, then infuse with NaCl via infusion pump and monitor cavernosal pressure.
   Normal intra-cavernosal pressure: >90 mm Hg
   Normal infusion to maintain erection: <20 mL/min
   Flow to maintain >20 mL/min = veno-occlusive dysfunction

TREATMENT

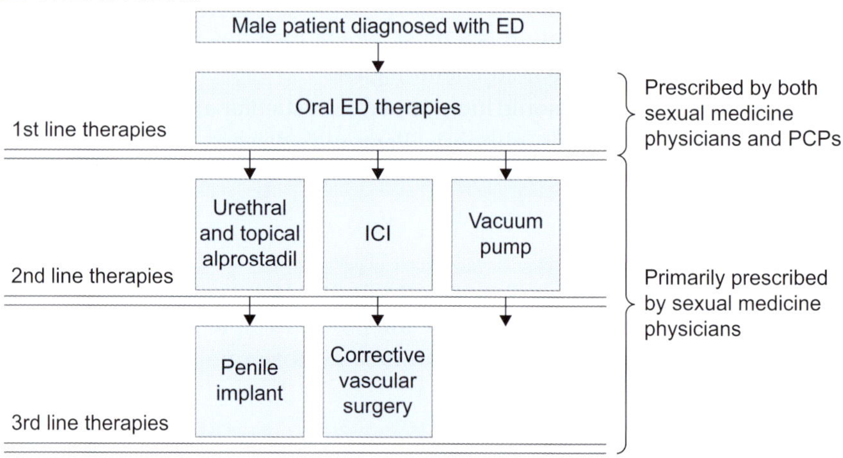

Current treatment approaches for erectile dysfunction (Konstantinos Hatzimouratidis).

Oral Drugs

- Sildenafil citrate
  - Doses of 25, 50, and 100 mg (on-demand).
  - Adverse effects: Headache, flushing, dyspepsia, and nasal congestion.

- Tadalafil
  - *Doses:* 2.5 and 5 mg (daily use) and 10 and 20 mg (on demand).
  - Adverse effects: Back pain, myalgia, headache, flushing, dyspepsia, and nasal congestion.
- Vardenafil
  - *Doses:* Film-coated 5, 10 and 20 mg and oro-dispersible tablet at 10 mg.
  - *Adverse effects:* Headache, flushing, dyspepsia, and nasal congestion.
- Avanafil
  - *Doses:* 50, 100, and 200 mg (on-demand).
  - *Adverse effects:* Headache and flushing.
- Udenafil
  - *Doses:* 100 and 200 mg (on-demand).
  - *Adverse effects:* Headache, flushing, dyspepsia, and nasal congestion.

Intracavernosal Injection Therapy (Self-administered)

An ultrathin needle (27–30 g) is used to inject the drug into the corpora cavernosa on the lateral aspect (3 or 9 o'clock).

Alprostadil (PGE1) (Monomix)

Alprostadil is the only drug approved for IC injections worldwide.

Doses: 1–40 mg and 60 mg (in some cases).

Mechanism of action: The effect is mediated through prostaglandin E receptors targeting membrane-bound adenylyl cyclase, thus increasing cAMP and α-adrenoceptor-mediated inhibition of noradrenaline release, causing both vasodilatation and veno-occlusion

Papaverine

Doses: 7.5–15 mg.

Papaverine-phentolamine (Bi-Mix)

Doses: Papaverine hydrochloride (15 mg/mL) and phentolamine mesylate (0.5 mg/mL) in a 2-mL ampoule (commercial preparation).

Papaverine-phentolamine-PGE1 (Tri-Mix)

Doses - Papaverine 17.64 mg + phentolamine 0.58 mg + PGE1 5.8 mg

Intraurethral Alprostadil as Muse (Medicated Urethral System for Erection)

After voiding, a small applicator is passed through the meatus and a single dose of alprostadil is injected into the urethral mucosa.

Doses: 125, 250, 500, and 1,000 mg.

Vacuum Erectile Device

A vacuum pump can be used alone or along with oral medications or intracavernosal injection with vasoactive drugs.

Method: Penis is placed in a plastic cylinder made airtight using a lubricant cream, and then is pressed against the pubic bone. Once an erection is achieved, a rubber constriction ring is slipped onto the base of the penis, thus preventing venous drainage and detumescence.

Surgical Treatment

Penile Implants (Penile Prostheses)

Two types: Malleable (bendable) or inflatable/hydraulic.

1. *Malleable:* Consists of a pair of malleable rods surgically placed into the two corpora cavernosa. During the sexual act, the implant needs to be lifted by hand to the erect position for insertion.
2. *Inflatable:* 2 types: 2-piece and 3-piece.

Consists of 2 inflatable cylinders placed into the cavernous bodies, connected through tubes to a fluid-filled reservoir, which is implanted in the Retzius space or intra-abdominally between the bowels and a pump placed in an artificially created subcutaneous space into the scrotum.

For inflation, the pump is squeezed 10–15 times, letting the fluid travel from the reservoir into the cylinders, and the patient can feel an erection. After completion of sex, the deflation valve opens and the fluid returns to the reservoir, and the penis returns to a flaccid state.

This process does not interfere with the sensation on the skin, orgasm, ejaculation or fertility of the male.

Vascular Surgery on the Penis

Penile revascularization procedures are performed for arterial insufficiency and/or veno-occlusive disease.

An isolated inferior epigastric artery is anastomosed to penile vessels, and/or resection of abnormal vein(s) can be done.

KEY POINTS

- Erectile dysfunction is best described as a lifestyle disease.
- To prevent its progression, the most effective approach is to reduce sugar, salt, smoking, alcohol, and an inactive lifestyle, and to improve sleep.
- Available treatments are effective but only provide temporary relief, and the condition may recur.
- Once ED develops, it serves as a warning sign of impending vascular disease.
- ED also has a psychological component, so patients' partners should be supportive.

SUGGESTED READING

1. Hackett G, Kirby M, Wylie K, Heald A, Ossei-Gerning N, Edwards D, et al. British Society for Sexual Medicine guidelines on the management of erectile dysfunction in men—2017. The journal of sexual medicine. 2018;15(4):430-57.
2. Hatzimouratidis K, Salonia A, Adaikan G, Buvat J, Carrier S, El-Meliegy A, et al. Pharmacotherapy for erectile dysfunction: recommendations from the Fourth International Consultation for Sexual Medicine (ICSM 2015). The Journal of Sexual Medicine. 2016;13(4):465-88.
3. Kirana PS, Tripodi F, Reisman Y, Porst H. The EFS and ESSM syllabus of clinical sexology. Amsterdam, the Netherlands: Medix; 2013.
4. Kirby M. The circle of lifestyle and erectile dysfunction. Sexual Medicine Reviews. 2015;3(3):169-82.
5. Latini DM, Penson DF, Wallace KL, Lubeck DP, Lue TF. Clinical and psychosocial characteristics of men with erectile dysfunction: Baseline data from ExCEED™. The Journal of Sexual Medicine. 2006;3(6):1059-67.
6. Liu CC, Huang SP, Wu WJ, Lee YC, Wang CJ. Management of erectile dysfunction with hypogonadism. Urological Science. 2010;21(3):113-7.
7. Liu Q, Zhang Y, Wang J, Li S, Cheng Y, Guo J, et al. Erectile dysfunction and depression: a systematic review and meta-analysis. The Journal of Sexual Medicine. 2018;15(8):1073-82.
8. Mallepalli PK, Vanamali DR, Raghuram M, Reddy S. An approach to the assessment of a patient with erectile dysfunction. Archives of Mental Health. 2014;15(1):32-7.
9. Montorsi P, Ravagnani PM, Galli S, Briganti A, Salonia A, Dehò F, et al. Association between erectile dysfunction and coronary artery disease: a case report study. The Journal of Sexual Medicine. 2005;2(4):575-82.
10. Nguyen HM, Gabrielson AT, Hellstrom WJ. Erectile dysfunction in young men—a review of the prevalence and risk factors. Sexual Medicine Reviews. 2017;5(4):508-20.
11. Xu Y, Zhang Y, Yang Y, Liu L, Chen Y, Liu X. Prevalence and correlates of erectile dysfunction in type 2 diabetic men: a population-based cross-sectional study in Chinese men. International Journal of Impotence Research. 2019;31(1):9-14.

10 CHAPTER

Premature Ejaculation

Percy B Kharas

INTRODUCTION

Premature ejaculation (PE) is the most common male sexual dysfunction, characterized by ejaculation that occurs sooner than desired during partnered sexual activity.

It is defined by three key dimensions:

1. A short ejaculatory latency time.
2. A perceived lack of ejaculatory control.
3. Negative personal consequences such as distress, frustration, or the avoidance of sexual intimacy.

Treatment typically involves a multi modal approach combining behavioral, psychological, and pharmacological therapies.

CLINICAL ASPECTS: DEFINITION AND CLASSIFICATION

The International Society of Sexual Medicine (ISSM) Recognizes four types of PE, which differ in their causes and treatment approaches:

1. *Lifelong (primary) PE:* Ejaculation that has always occurred before or within approximately 1 minute of Vaginal Penetration since the first sexual encounter. It is often linked to Genetic and Neurobiological factors.
2. *Acquired (secondary) PE:* A clinically significant reduction in ejaculatory latency that develops after a period of normal ejaculatory function. An Intravaginal Ejaculatory Latency Time (IELT) of 3 minutes or less is common. It is often associated with Psychological Factors or other medical issues like Erectile Dysfunction (ED).
3. *Natural Variable PE:* Occasional and Irregular Episodes of Rapid Ejaculation, often due to situational factors like stress, a new partner, or infrequent sexual activity. It is not a formal sexual dysfunction and is best managed with reassurance & psychoeducation.
4. *Premature-like Ejaculatory Dysfunction:* A patient's subjective complain of PE, despite an actual IELT that is within or even longer than the normal range.

CAUSES AND ASSOCIATED FACTORS

Premature ejaculation is a complex condition influenced by a combination of psychological and biological elements.

- *Psychological:* Performance Anxiety, Stress, Depression, low self-esteem, poor body image, and relationship problems are frequently associated with PE. These issues can create a negative cycle, with PE causing psychological distress, that in turn increases the problem.
- *Biological:* Severe biological factors are implicated, particularly in lifelong PE:
- *Neurobiological:* Imbalances in the brain's serotonin levels play a significant role.
- Low serotonin neurotransmission is linked to a lower ejaculatory threshold.
- *Genetics:* Some research suggests a genetic predisposition to a lifelong PE.

Comorbidities: Acquired PE can be associated with other conditions, including ED, prostatitis, and hyperthyroidism. Men with ED may rush to ejaculate fearing the loss of their erection.

EVALUATION

- *History taking:* Clinical History is Crucial. Elicit the Patient's and Partner's Perspective on the Problem.
- *Intravaginal Ejaculatory Latency Time (IELT):* The estimated time from vaginal penetration to ejaculation. 1 minute or less for lifelong PE, and 3 minutes or less for Acquired PE, is the Common Criterion.
- *Perceived Control:* The man's ability or inability to delay ejaculation.
- *Distress/Bother:* Negative Consequences. Anxiety, Frustration, No Sexual Intimacy, etc.
- *Sexual History:* Frequency of sexual activity and masturbation.
- *Presence of ED:* PE secondary to maintaining an erection.
- Partner's sexual health and response. The impact of relationship on PE.
- *Medical and Psychological History:* Chronic Diseases—e.g., Diabetes, Thyroid Problems.

NEUROLOGICAL PROBLEMS AND INJURIES

- Psychological issues.
- Current medications or substance abuse.
- *Relevant past experiences:* Strict religious upbringing, past sexual trauma.
- *Questionnaires:* Premature Ejaculation Diagnostic Tools (PEDT): To objectively assess severity and impact.

PHYSICAL EXAMINATION

To identify or Rule out the causes of acquired PE.

- *General Physical Examination:* Assessment of overall health. Vital Information—Pulse, BP. Palpation Auscultation. Secondary Sexual Characters—Endocrine Dysfunction, e.g., Gynecomastia.

- *Genitourinary Examination:* Penis, Scrotal Sac Organs for Anatomical/ Pathological Problems.
- *Neurological Assessment:* Lower Limbs and Genital Area.
- *Digital Rectal Exam:* Prostatitis-Painful Ejaculation.

INVESTIGATION

- Lab and diagnostic tests are generally not performed routinely for PE, unless the history or examination suggests an underlying Medical Cause.
- *Routine Lab Tests:* As Needed.
  - *Hormone Testing:* Ser. testosterone, prolactin
- *Thyroid hormones:* It may be checked if Pt. also presents with ED, low libido, or symptoms suggestive of hormonal imbalance.
  - *Urine analysis/culture:* If UTI/Prostatitis Suspected.
  - *Neurological tests:* Nerve Conduction Studies in rare case where indicated.
- The Diagnostic Process is sometimes very important to Guide Appropriate Treatment.

MANAGEMENT STRATEGIES

An individualized multimodal treatment plan is generally the most effective approach for managing PE.

Behavioral and Psychological Therapies

- *Psychoeducation and counseling:* Therapy often involving the partner, can help address anxiety, relationship issues, and unrealistic expectations.
- *The " Stop-Start" Technique:* The man or his partner stimulates the penis until the man feels the sensation of imminent ejaculation. Stimulation is than stopped until the sensation subsides. This is repeated three or four times before allowing ejaculation.
- *The "Squeeze" Technique:* Similar to the stop- start method, but just before ejaculation, the man or his partner squeezes the tip of the penis to temporarily decrease arousal and postpone ejaculation.

Pelvic Floor Exercises (Kegels)

Strengthening the pelvic floor muscles can improve ejaculatory control. Men can find these muscles by stopping urination mod stream. The exercise involves tightening and holding these muscles for a few seconds, repeating in sets.

PHARMACOLOGICAL THERAPIES

- *Topical Anesthetics:* Creams or sprays containing numbing agents like lidocaine or prilocaine can be applied to the penis 10–15 minutes before intercourse to reduce sensation. Use of a condom is recommended to prevent transference and numbness in the partner.

- *Selective Serotonin Reuptake Inhibitors (SSRI's):* Of label use of daily SSRI's such as paroxetine, sertraline, or fluoxetine, is a common and effective treatment. These medications are a gold standard for PE due to their side effect of delaying ejaculation.
- *Dapoxetine:* A short-acting SSRI specifically developed and approved in many countries for on demand treatment of PE. It is taken 1–3 hours before sexual activity.
- *Tricyclic Antidepressants (TCA's):* Clomipramine is an antidepressant that is also used off-label to delay ejaculation.
- *Tramadol:* This opioid analgesic can delay ejaculation but it is reserved for refractory cases due to the risk of addiction. I should not be combined with SSRI's due to the risk of serotonin syndrome.
- *PDE5 Inhibitors (Sildenafil and Tadalafil):* These are primarily for treating erectile dysfunction but can be used in combination with SSRI's for men with co-existing ED and PE. They do not directly delay ejaculation but can reduce performance anxiety and improve control perception.

Combination Therapy

Evidence suggests that combining different treatment modalities often yields the best results.

For instance, combining a daily SSRI with behavioral techniques or counseling can improve long-term outcomes and reduce the likelihood of relapse.

SUGGESTED READING

1. Abdo CH. The Impact of Ejaculatory Dysfunction upon the sufferer and his partner. Transl Androl Urol. 2016;5(4):460-9.
2. Attallah S, Haydar A. Psychological Interventions & Discussion Approaches in Management of PE. Arab J Urol. 2021.
3. Butcher M, Zubert T. Topical Agents for PE. A Review. Sex Med Rev. 2020;8(1):92-9.
4. EL-Hamd MA, Saleh R. Premature Ejaculation: An Update. Asian J Androl. 2019;21(5):425-32.
5. Howton K, Catalan J, Martin P, Fagg J. Long Term Outcome of Sex. Behav Res Ther. 1986;24(6):665-75.
6. McCabe MP, Balon R. Consensus Statements from the International Consultation on Sexual Medicine 2021. J Sex Med. 2022.
7. Puppo V. Puppo G. Comprehensive Review of the Physiology of Male Ejaculation: Premature ejaculation is not a disease. Clin Anat. 2016;29(1):111-9.
8. Raveendran AV, Agarwal A. PE Current Concepts in Management: A narrative review. Int J Reprod Biomed. 2021;19(1):5-22.
9. Sansone A, Aversa A, Corona G, Fisher AD, Isidori AM, La Vignera S, et al. Management of PE A Clinical Guideline from the Italian Soc. of Andrology & Sexual Medicine. Endocrinol Invest. 2021;44(5):1103-18.
10. Wu T, Yue X, Duan X, Luo D, Cheng Y, Tian Y, et al. Efficacy and Safety of Medications for PE: A Systemic Review & Meta Analysis. Urology. 2012;80(3):618-24.

11 CHAPTER

Sexual History Taking: A Comprehensive Guidelines

Vaidehi Thakur, Deep Kamal

INTRODUCTION

Sexual health is not merely the absence of disease; it is a state of physical, emotional, mental, and social well-being in relation to sexuality. It profoundly impacts an individual's overall quality of life. Consequently, taking a sexual history must be a routine component of comprehensive health care, not reserved only for situations with clinical features suggestive of sexually transmitted infections. This thorough process is essential, as it enables the clinician to provide high-quality patient care by appropriately assessing and screening individuals for a broad range of sexual health concerns, ultimately leading to a comprehensive and accurate diagnosis.

CREATING THE CLINICAL ENVIRONMENT AND COMMUNICATION

Sexual History Taking

The cornerstone of a successful sexual history is a welcoming, safe, and non-judgmental clinical environment starting at Registration.

- Clinician must foster inclusivity by establishing the patient's name, preferred pronouns, and Sexual Orientation and Gender Identity (SOGI). Explicit consent is mandatory before proceeding.
- *Gender Identity is separate from sexual orientation; determine it via a two-step process:* Sex assigned at birth and current gender identity (e.g., transgender, gender diverse). This deliberate approach validates the patient and ensures accurate communication.

Putting the Patient at Ease

Many patients feel uncomfortable discussing sexual history due to past abuse or trauma.

- Clinicians must normalize the process, assuring patients it's a standard, important part of routine care. For acute discomfort, offering all testing options upfront may be best.
- Ensure absolute privacy and confidentiality, clarifying limits (e.g., immediate danger). The clinician's role is to put the patient at ease, find the real problem, gather history, and collaboratively develop a management plan.

General Communication Skills

Clinician presentation and speech are as vital as the questions asked.

- Maintain a professional attitude and a clear self-introduction.
- Be consistently cool, polite, and strictly nonjudgmental. Neutral expression and tone are paramount.
- Be conscious of your body language; it should convey openness and attentiveness (e.g., maintaining appropriate eye contact, avoiding crossed arms).
- Where appropriate and consented, inquire about the history of both partners to understand the transmission dynamics.
- Ensure privacy and confidentiality throughout the entire encounter.

BASIC HISTORY AND INITIATION

Basic History Notes

Before moving to the sexual history, record the essential demographic and background details for context:

- *Demographics:* Name, age, sex (as identified by the patient), and address.
- *Social Context:* Religion, marital status, occupation, education, and contact details.
- *Background:* Information about other family members, and a full review of *Past, Personal, Family, Medical, Surgical, and Obstetric history*. Any chronic illness (e.g., diabetes, hypertension) or previous surgery can impact sexual function.

Initiating the Sexual History

Permission must be asked directly and politely:

- *"May I ask you a few questions about your sexual health and sexual practices? I understand that these questions are personal, but they are important for your overall health"*
- *Alternatively: "At this point in the visit, I will ask some questions regarding your sexual life. Will that be ok?"*

Guiding Principles

- Ask these questions to all patients, regardless of age, gender, or marital status. Sexual health is relevant across the lifespan.
- Emphasize that these questions are as important as questions about other areas of your physical and mental health.
- Reiterate that this information is kept in strict confidence unless you or someone else is being hurt or is in danger.
- Utilize a *preconsultation questionnaire* if appropriate, as some patients prefer to write down sensitive details before speaking to them aloud.

TABLE 1: Monash women's health program female sexuality satisfaction questionnaire.

Question	*Option 1*	*Option 2*	*Option 3*
1. I have had sexual activity within the last 24 hours	Not at all	Once	More than once
2. My sexual activity involved a partner	Yes (continue)	No (Go to Q6)	
3. My sexual activity involved intercourse	Yes	No	
4. I initiated the sexual encounter	Yes (Go to Q6)	No	
5. My partner initiated sex	Yes (continue)	No	
5b. I was receptive (I was ready or willing to receive favorably)	Not at all	Moderately so	Very much so
6. I become easily aroused	Not at all	Moderately so	Very much so
7. My vaginal lubrication (wetness) was	Absent	Adequate	A great deal
8. I had an orgasm during sexual activity	Yes	No	
9. I achieve orgasm	With great difficulty	With some effort	Very easily
10. My sexual experience was	Not pleasurable	Moderately pleasurable	Extremely pleasurable
11. I found sex satisfying	Not at all	Moderately so	Very much so

- *Always conclude the initiation by asking: Do you have any questions or concerns about your sexual health before we get started?*

Preconsultation Questionnaire

Table 1 shows Monash Women's Health Program.

Please answer the questions shown in **Table 1** in terms of your experience in the last 24 hours.

Please read each statement carefully and mark the appropriate box with an X corresponding to the extent each statement applied to you.

All questions need to be answered if you engaged in sexual activity in the last 24 hours.

Table 2 shows sexual health inventory for men.

Questioning Techniques and Terminology

The clinician must skillfully transition between different questioning styles:

- *Open Questioning:* Used to define the core complaint and encourage narrative. Examples: "*How can I help you?,*" "*What is the problem?,*" or "*What do you think caused the difficulty?*"

TABLE 2: The international index of erectile function (iief-5): sexual health inventory for men (SHIM).

Name			***Date***		
Sexual Health Questionnaire: Answer the sexual health questions by circling your answer and adding up your score.					
	1	***2***	***3***	***4***	***5***
1. Rate your confidence in your ability to get and keep an erection?	Very Low	Low	Moderate	High	Very High
2. When you have an erection with sexual stimulation, how often are your erections hard enough for penetration?	Almost never or never	A few times	Sometimes	Most times	Almost always or always
3. During sexual intercourse, how often are you able to maintain your erection during penetration?	Almost never or never	A few times	Sometimes	Most times	Almost always or always
4. During sexual intercourse, has it been difficult to maintain your erection to completion of intercourse?	Extremely difficult	Very difficult	Difficult	Slightly difficult	Not difficult
5. When attempting sexual intercourse, how often is it satisfactory for you?	Almost never or never	A few times	Sometimes	Most times	Almost always or always
Total score: The Sexual Health Inventory for Men (SHIM) classifies ED severity with the following breakpoints:					
1–7: Severe ED	8–11: Moderate ED		12–16: Mild–moderate ED	17–21: Mild ED 22–25: No ED	
6. *Check any ED treatments you have tried:* ☐ Pills/Medication ☐ Vacuum Device ☐ Injection Therapy ☐ MUSE™ ☐ Other					

- *Closed Questioning:* Used for specific, factual data. Examples: "*Have you had this problem before?*" (Expects a specific reply: YES/NO).
- *Finding out the Problem:* Requires careful and tactful elucidation. Avoid judgmental or loaded words like "Impotence" or "Frigidity". Any vagueness must be clarified immediately (e.g., "When you say 'things are slow,' what specifically do you mean?")
- *Choice of Terminology:* Decide whether to use vernacular terms OR medical terms in discussion. The use of certain street versions or common

colloquialisms may assume a very relaxed and empathic discussion, but the clinician must gauge the patient's comfort. Clarity and patient preference should always govern the choice of words.

Core Sexual Concerns and Evaluation

- *Detail:* Assess Desire, Arousal, Penetration, Ejaculation, Orgasm and Pain. Ask regarding Detail Onset, Duration, Severity, Progress, Aggravating, Relieving, and Associated factors.
- *Context:* Interpret within a biopsychosocial framework: Sexual Identity, Health status, Relationship factors, Culture, and Expectations.

THE 5 'P'S FRAMEWORK

The *5 'P's framework* is a highly effective, structured method for taking a *sexual behavior history*. The ultimate goal of the 5Ps is to improve patient health by facilitating full disclosure of sexual practices, especially in patients who may initially be uncomfortable.

Partners

- Are you currently having sex of any kind? (Oral, vaginal, or anal).
- If no, have you ever had sex of any kind with another person? (This ensures history is taken even if they are not currently active).
- In recent months, how many sex partners have you had?
- What is/are the gender(s) of your sex partner(s)?
- Do you or your partner(s) currently have other sex partners (non-monogamy)?

Practices

- Explain the need for specific questions to assess STI risk, as different tests are used for different body parts involved in sex.
- What kind of sexual contact do you have?
  - Do you have genital sex (penis in the vagina)?
  - Anal sex (penis in the anus)? Are you a top and/or bottom?
  - Oral sex (mouth on penis, vagina, or anus)?
- Do you meet your partners online or through apps?
- Have you or any of your partners used drugs in conjunction with sex?
- Have you exchanged sex for your needs (money, housing, drugs, etc.)?

Protection from STIs

- Do you and your partner(s) discuss STI prevention?
- If you use prevention tools, what methods do you use? (Male or female condoms, etc.).
- *How often do you use this method(s)? Be specific about:*

- Frequencies (e.g., "always," "half the time") and Times they do not use a method (e.g., "never with my main partner," or "only when drinking").
- Have you received HPV, hepatitis A, and/or hepatitis B shots?
- Are you aware of PEP (Post-Exposure Prophylaxis), a medicine that can prevent HIV? Have you ever used it or considered using it?

Past History of STIs

- *Have you ever been tested for STIs and HIV? (Offer testing:* Would you like to be tested?).
- Have you been diagnosed with an STI in the past? When? Did you get treatment?
- Have you had any symptoms that keep coming back?
- Has your current or any former partners ever been diagnosed or treated for an STI?
- Were you tested for the same STI(s) your partner had?
- Do you know your partner(s) HIV status?

Key STI Prevention Strategies to Highlight

- Not having sex (Abstinence).
- Mutual monogamy with a tested, uninfected partner.
- Using PEP or PrEP (Pre-Exposure Prophylaxis).
- Using condoms the right way every time a person has sex.

Pregnancy Prevention

- Do you think you would like to have children at some point? When do you think that might be?
- How important is it to you to prevent pregnancy (until then)?
- Are you or your partner using contraception or practicing any form of birth control?
- Would you like to talk about ways to prevent pregnancy? Do you need any information on birth control?

FINAL TOUCH-UP AND MANAGEMENT PLAN

Closing Consultation

To finalize the consultation, summarize the key points for mutual understanding and reaffirm confidentiality. Conclude by thanking the patient for their openness and encouraging any protective practices they currently employ.

Finally, ask a concluding question: "What other concerns or questions regarding your sexual health or practices would you like to discuss?" During this wrap-up, gently inquire about any history of trauma, sexual abuse, or violence. Also, be sure to consider asking about sexual functioning, including pleasure and performance, and refer for care as needed.

Agreeing on a Management Plan

The Management Plan requires patient agreement through a collaborative discussion, fostering a partnership with the doctor. This ensures better treatment adherence. Patient consent may permit involving a partner in specific cases like couples counselling or STI planning.

TAKE-HOME MESSAGE

Effective sexual history taking requires a foundation of non-judgmental respect and privacy. By actively establishing a safe environment, confirming identity, gaining explicit consent, and normalizing the inquiry, clinicians build the necessary trust. Using structured techniques like the 5 'P's (Partners, Practices, Protection, Past STIs, Pregnancy Prevention) ensures a comprehensive assessment of risk and function. The final step involves a collaborative management plan, ensuring the patient is an empowered partner in their care. A good sexual history is not just about finding disease; it's about providing holistic, preventative, and patient-centered care that honors the complexity of human sexuality.

SUGGESTED READING

1. Althof SE, Rosen RC, Symonds T, Mundayat R, May K, Abraham L, et al. The development and validation of a new questionnaire to assess sexual satisfaction in men: the Sexual Satisfaction Scale for Men (SSS-M). BJU Int. 2005;95(8):1244-9.
2. American Medical Association. Principles of Medical Ethics. Chicago: American Medical Association; 2001.
3. Basson R, Berman J, Burnett A, Derogatis L, Ferguson D, Fourcroy J, et al. Report of the international consensus development conference on female sexual dysfunction: definitions and classifications. J Urol. 2000;163(3):888-93.
4. Canadian guidelines for sexual health education. Sex Information and Education Council of Canada (SIECCAN). [updated 2019; cited 2025 Dec 22]. Available from: http://sieccan.org/wp-content/uploads/2021/02/ SIECCANCanadian-GuidelinesforSexualHealthEduca tion1.pdf
5. Carmona C, Crutwell J, Burnham M, Polak L. Shared decision-making: summary of NICE guidance . BMJ. 2021;373 :n1430.
6. Centres for Disease Control and Prevention. A Guide to Taking a Sexual History. Atlanta: CDC; 2017.
7. Centres for Disease Control and Prevention. Recommendations for the laboratory-based screening of sexually transmitted diseases. Atlanta: CDC; 2014
8. Centres for Disease Control and Prevention. Taking a Sexual History: Practical Tips. Atlanta: CDC; 2017.
9. Davison SL, Bell RJ, La China M, Holden SL, Davis SR. Assessing sexual function in well women: Validity and reliability of the Monash Women's Health Program Female Sexual Satisfaction Questionnaire. The journal of sexual medicine. 2008;5(11):2575-86.

10. Goldfarb A, Pukall CF. The diagnosis and management of female sexual pain. CMAJ. 2016;188(17-18):1244-50.
11. Hinchliff S, Gott M, Partridge M. Taking a sexual history. Br J Nurs. 2005;14(16): 869-73.
12. National LGBTQIA+ Health Education Center. A guide for collecting data on sexual orientation and gender identity. [updated 2022; cited 2025 Dec 20]. Available from: https://www.lgbtqiahealtheducation.org/wp-content/uploads/2022/05/TFIE-64_Updates2022_ReadySetGo_10_18_22.pdf
13. Neighbour R. The Inner Consultation: How to Develop an Effective and Enjoyable Clinical Practice. USA: CRC Press; 2004.
14. NHS Health Scotland. Sexual Health Standards for Primary Care. Scotland: NHS Health; 2011.
15. Poteat T, German D, Kerrigan D. Managing sexuality in the context of health care: A qualitative study of transgender women. Qual Health Res. 2013;23(7):905-18.
16. Rosen RC, Riley A, Wagner G, Osterloh IH, Kirkpatrick J, Mishra A. The international index of erectile function (IIEF): a multidimensional scale for assessment of erectile dysfunction. Urology. 1997;49(6):822-30.
17. World Health Organization. Sexual health. [2025; cited 2025 Dec 21]. Available from: https://www.who.int/health-topics/sexual-health#tab=tab_1

12 CHAPTER

Sexuality and Gen Z: The Paradigmatic Shift in Modern Human Connection—A Sexual Medicine Perspective

Naisargi Patel

INTRODUCTION: GEN Z AND THE DIGITAL SEXUAL LANDSCAPE

Generation Z is characterized by high technological literacy, global connectivity, and unprecedented access to information. Unlike previous cohorts, Gen Z navigates romantic and sexual relationships within a digital ecosystem, where social media platforms, dating apps, and online communities shape perceptions of attraction, intimacy, and consent. These digital tools provide both opportunities and challenges: they allow for exploration of sexual identity, orientation and social connection but can also facilitate risk behaviors, emotional burnout, and unrealistic relationship expectations.

From a clinical perspective, this digital immersion requires practitioners to understand how online behaviors influence sexual development, risk-taking, and relationship satisfaction. Clinicians must integrate knowledge of social media dynamics, digital communication, and emerging sexual norms into counseling and health promotion strategies.

CONCEPTUALIZING SEXUALITY IN GEN Z

Sexuality includes biological sex, gender identity, sexual orientation, sexual behavior, and interpersonal intimacy. Gen Z demonstrates a nuanced understanding of these dimensions, with growing recognition of fluid and non-binary identities. The language of sexual identity has expanded to include terms such as pansexual, demisexual, gray sexual, and non-binary, reflecting increased societal acceptance and individual self-expression.

For sexual medicine practitioners, recognizing these identities is crucial for delivering culturally competent care. This includes providing affirming sexual health counseling, addressing reproductive health needs, and reducing stigma and taboo in clinical interactions.

SEXUAL BEHAVIOR TRENDS AND RELATIONSHIP MODELS

Gen Z relationships often deviate from traditional monogamous or long-term paradigms. Emerging trends include:

- *Situationships:* Undefined relationships with ambiguous boundaries

- *Talking stage:* Preliminary dating via digital communication
- *Cuffing season:* Seasonal short-term partnerships
- *Digital breakup behaviors:* Ghosting and benching (Fortune, 2023; The Karan Blog, 2024)

While these practices may seem casual, many Gen Z individuals value emotional transparency, mutual respect, and consent. Clinicians should consider these patterns when discussing sexual health, relationship satisfaction, and emotional well-being with patients.

Sexual experimentation, facilitated by digital exposure, also raises clinical considerations for sexually transmitted infections (STIs), unintended pregnancies, and consent education. Evidence suggests that Gen Z demonstrates increased sexual awareness but also engages in higher-risk behaviors online, emphasizing the need for comprehensive sexual education and clinical guidance.

TECHNOLOGY, SOCIAL MEDIA, AND SEXUAL EXPRESSION

Digital media serves as both a medium and a challenge in Gen Z sexuality. Dating applications (Tinder, Bumble, Hinge) provide access to diverse partners and facilitate identity exploration. However, algorithmic biases, curated profiles, and immediate feedback loops contribute to superficial evaluations, emotional fatigue, and relationship anxiety.

Gen Z generation who use Instagram frequently are more prone to engage in sexual behavior and drug abuse. IJMER 2023 study shows exposure to sexual and substance related content on Instagram likely to harm Gen Z' sexual and drug related behaviors.

Digital Body Language (DBL)—such as emoji usage, typing speed, and message patterns—has become an essential medium through which Gen Z express and interprets interest and attraction. Clinicians should incorporate discussions about online behaviors into sexual health counseling, including the psychological impact of digital rejection, pressure to maintain online personalities, and consent in virtual sexual interactions.

MENTAL HEALTH, CONSENT, AND SELF-LOVE

Mental health is important to healthy sexual development among Gen Z. Anxiety, depression, and emotional burnout are increased by social comparison, FOMO (fear of missing out), and constant online engagement. Consequently, Gen Z prioritizes self-care, emotional intelligence, and boundary setting in sexual relationships.

Clinically, this shift highlights the importance of integrating mental health assessment into sexual medicine consultations. Open dialogue about boundaries, enthusiastic consent, and emotional readiness can enhance sexual satisfaction and reduce adverse outcomes.

CLINICAL IMPLICATIONS AND SEXUAL HEALTH PRACTICE

Understanding Gen Z sexuality informs several areas of clinical practice:

- *Comprehensive Sexual Health Counseling:* Clinicians must discuss safe sexual practices, contraceptive options, STI prevention, and consent in ways that acknowledge fluid identities.
- *Affirming Care:* Recognize and validate diverse sexual orientations and gender identities to reduce stigma and improve patient engagement.
- *Digital Education:* Address risks and responsibilities associated with online sexual interactions, including sexting, image-sharing, and dating apps.
- *Emotional Well-being:* Incorporate mental health screening and counseling into sexual medicine visits, emphasizing self-love and boundary-setting as part of sexual health.
- *Tailored Interventions:* Adapt interventions to the unique relational patterns of Gen Z, including non-traditional relationships, polyamory, and situational arrangements.

  These approaches enable clinicians to provide holistic, evidence-based care that addresses both physical and psychosocial aspects of sexual health.

PARADIGMATIC SHIFT IN SEXUALITY

The shift observed in Gen Z represents a paradigmatic transformation in sexual norms. Unlike previous generations, Gen Z views sexuality as fluid, relational, and self-defined rather than rigid or prescriptive. The integration of digital media, global cultural exposure, and mental health awareness has accelerated the acceptance of diverse sexual expressions and practices.

From a sexual medicine standpoint, this transformation necessitates adaptation in clinical frameworks, moving from a purely biomedical model to a biopsychosocial model that incorporates identity, technology, and emotional health.

FUTURE DIRECTIONS AND RECOMMENDATIONS

As Gen Z matures, sexual medicine practice must evolve to address:

- Emerging sexual technologies (telehealth, AI-assisted sexual education, virtual reality intimacy)
- Intersectionality of sexual identity, culture, and mental health
- Evidence-based guidelines for managing digital sexual behaviors and emotional well-being
- Policy-level interventions to ensure comprehensive sex education is accessible and inclusive.
- Clinicians are encouraged to maintain continuous education on evolving trends, engage in culturally competent practice, and advocate for inclusive sexual health education policies.

KEY POINTS

- Gen Z views sexuality as fluid, inclusive, and identity-driven.
- Digital interactions significantly influence sexual behavior, relationship formation, and consent practices.
- Mental health and sexual well-being are interconnected; anxiety and social media pressures affect sexual decision-making.
- Affirming care and inclusive language improve engagement and reduce stigma in sexual medicine practice.
- Comprehensive counseling should address safer sexual behaviors, consent, relational dynamics, and emotional intelligence.

SUGGESTED READING

1. Appinio. (2024). Gen Z dating insights in the US. US: Appinio Research; 2024.
2. Better Health Victoria. (2022). Sexuality explained. [online] Available from https://www.betterhealth.vic.gov.au [Last accessed January, 2026].
3. Fortune. (2023, May 12). Are teenagers having sex? CDC Gen Z situationships & sneaky links. [online] Available from https://fortune.com [Last accessed January, 2026].
4. ICMR. (2023). Youth sexual and reproductive health in India: Emerging trends. India: Indian Council of Medical Research; 2023.
5. Indigo Therapy Group. (2025). Gen Z dating: How the youngest generation is changing the game. [online] Available from https://indigotherapygroup.com [Last accessed January, 2025].
6. Kanhar K, Kumar L. IJMER (2023) – Impact of sexuality and substance abuse on Generation Z with reference to Instagram. IJMER. 2023;4(5):12.
7. Karan Blog. (2024). Understanding 10 Gen Z relationship terms. [online] Available from https://www.thekaran.in/blog [Last accessed January, 2026].
8. Logopsycom. (2023). Inclusive and comprehensive sexual education for Generation Z. [online] Available from https://logopsycom.com [Last accessed January, 2026].
9. McKinsey & Company. (2023). What is Gen Z? [online] Available from https://www.mckinsey.com [Last accessed January, 2026].
10. My Wellbeing. (2024). Generation Z, social media and its impact on romantic relationships. [online] Available from https://mywellbeing.com [Last accessed January, 2026].
11. NACO. (2023). National adolescent sexual and reproductive health program: Annual report. National AIDS Control Organization[online] Available from https://naco.gov.in/documentsreports [Last accessed January, 2026].
12. NDTV. (2023). What is gray sexuality? Uncovering the latest trend sweeping Gen Z. [online] Available from https://www.ndtv.com [Last accessed January, 2026].
13. New Indian Express. (2025, Jan 16). Gen Z redefines love: New lingo, modern relationships, and evolving perspectives on commitment. [online] Available from https://www.newindianexpress.com [Last accessed January, 2026].
14. Partner Native. (2023). Gen Z relationships: A glimpse inside campus dating culture. Retrieved from https://partner.native.fm/blog/gen-z-relationships/
15. ResearchGate. (2022). Evolving label usage within Generation Z when self-describing sexual orientation. [online] Available from https://www.researchgate.net [Last accessed January, 2026].

16. SBU Online. (2024). Gen Z mental health. [online] Available from https://online.sbu.edu [Last accessed January, 2026].
17. UCDavis SHCS. (2023). Sexual communication and consent. [online] Available from https://shcs.ucdavis.edu [Last accessed January, 2026].
18. Vocal Media. (2024). The positive side of Gen Z love: Redefining relationships for a new era. [online] Available from https://vocal.media [Last accessed January, 2026].
19. WHO. (2022). Sexual and reproductive health for adolescents and youth. Geneva: World Health Organization; 2022.

13 CHAPTER

Age of Consent, Sex, and Where India Stands

Parul Saoji

INTRODUCTION

Sexual and reproductive health is vital to the holistic well-being of individuals, but it cannot be separated from legal, ethical and societal frameworks. One keystone in this domain is the concept of "age of consent"—the age at which a person is legally deemed capable of consenting to sexual activity. In India, the age of consent stands at 18 years. For gynecologists caring for adolescents, young adults and their families, understanding this law is critical: it affects medical decisions, confidentiality, reporting obligations, counseling, and the broader public health context.

This chapter aims to: (1) Review the legal evolution of the age of consent in India, (2) outline current law and its implications, (3) discuss the medical, ethical and public health aspects for gynecology practice, and (4) examine the debates and ways forward.

HISTORICAL EVOLUTION IN INDIA

The age of consent in India has undergone multiple changes, reflecting shifts in social norms, colonial legacy, child marriage practices and child-protection priorities. For instance:

- In 1860 under the original IPC, the age of consent for girls was just 10 years
- After the tragic case of 10-year-old Phulmoni Dasi who died following forced consummation of marriage, the colonial government passed the Age of Consent Act, 1891 raising the age to 12.
- Subsequently, the age rose to 14 in 1925, to 16 in 1940, and remained at 16 until 2012 for girls.
- With the enactment of POCSO, the age of consent for all genders was set at 18.

This evolution shows increasing recognition of adolescents' rights, changing societal attitudes toward child marriage and child sexual exploitation, and the shift from gender-specific definitions to more inclusive frameworks (i.e., covering all genders).

CURRENT LEGAL FRAMEWORK IN INDIA

Under the current statutes:

- The POCSO Act, 2012 defines a "child" as any person under 18 and criminalizes sexual activity with children.
- The Criminal Law (Amendment) Act, 2013 amended Section 375 of the IPC (which defines rape) to state that sexual intercourse with a person *below 18 years* of age is rape, even if consensual.
- The government has affirmed that the age of consent cannot be <18, and has opposed proposals to lower it.

KEY IMPLICATIONS

- Any sexual activity with someone under 18 years is punishable under child-sexual abuse laws, regardless of "consent" in the ordinary sense.
- There is currently *no* "close-in-age" (Romeo-&-Juliet) exception in Indian law.
- Marriage does *not* automatically legitimize sexual activity if one partner is under 18—sex with a child bride (below 18) is still criminalized under POCSO/IPC.

MEDICAL AND GYNECOLOGICAL IMPLICATIONS

As a practicing gynecologist, there are several areas where the age of consent (legal) and adolescent sexual/reproductive health intersects:

Consent vs. Capacity

From a clinical standpoint, adolescents may approach the clinic with sexual activity, contraceptive needs, pregnancy concerns or sexually transmitted infections. While medically we assess capacity, maturity and understanding, legally an individual under 18 cannot "consent" to sexual activity, so the clinician must be aware of reporting mandates and safeguarding protocols.

Confidentiality and Safeguarding

When an adolescent (<18) presents with sexual history, healthcare providers must balance confidentiality with legal obligations under POCSO (which requires reporting) and child protection. Knowing the legal age threshold helps guide when mandatory reporting may apply, and when to engage guardians, social services, or legal counsel.

Prevention of Adverse Outcomes of Early Sexual Activity

Adolescents engaging in sexual activity are at higher risk of unintended pregnancy, unsafe abortion, sexually transmitted infections (STIs), cervical/vaginal trauma, and psychosocial consequences. From a gynecology perspective: early sexual debut correlates with higher cervical cytological abnormalities later, higher risk of HPV infection and other complications. And early pregnancy carries increased obstetric risks (preterm delivery, low birth-weight, obstetric fistula in extreme cases). Thus, age of consent laws intersect with health promotion and preventive counseling.

Child Marriage and Its Effects

Child marriage is still present in parts of India, despite legal prohibition. The gynecologist often sees married adolescents (<18) with obstetric complications, menstrual issues, malnutrition and lack of autonomy. The legalizing of sexual activity below 18 (via marriage) remains a grey area; the law clearly criminalizes sex with under-18 even within marriage. A clinical lens demands that we be alert to marital status and age of partner, and advocate for delaying marriage and childbirth until biological and psychosocial maturity is achieved.

Education, Counseling, and Empowerment

Beyond clinical care, as gynecologists we have a public-health duty. Understanding legal thresholds enables us to provide age-appropriate sexual and reproductive health education, talk about consent, healthy relationships, contraception, STI prevention, and emotional readiness. We can work with schools, community organizations and parents to promote awareness of these legal and health aspects.

WHERE INDIA STANDS: CHALLENGES AND CONTRADICTIONS

Despite a robust legal framework, several challenges remain:

Legal-practice Gap

Although the law sets 18 as the age of consent, in practice many adolescents are sexually active earlier, and many marry under the legal age (child marriage). This creates a conflict between the lived reality and the legal ideal. For example, the law views sexual activity below 18 as abuse, but adolescents themselves may view their relationships as consensual.

Criminalization of Adolescent Relationships

Because there is no close-in-age exception, consensual sex between two adolescents (say 16 and 17) technically constitutes a crime. Critics argue this may hamper adolescents' access to healthcare (fear of reporting), or create perverse outcomes (e.g., under-reporting of sexual health concerns).

Mismatch Between Sexual Autonomy and Protection

Some scholars argue that while protecting children from exploitation is paramount, the blanket age-18 threshold may undermine adolescent autonomy and rights, particularly when the sexual activity is consensual and between peers.

Implementation and Awareness Issues

Many healthcare providers, educators and families lack clarity about the legal framework. Adolescents may not be aware of their rights, local services, or how the law intersects with health. In some regions, child marriage and early sexual debut persist due to poverty, gender inequality, cultural norms and low education levels.

FOR GYNECOLOGISTS: PRACTICAL GUIDANCE

Based on current law and clinical best practice, here are some actionable pointers for you as a gynecologist in India:

- *Know your legal thresholds:* Recognize that <18 years = minor for sexual consent. Keep up-to-date with state law and reporting obligations under POCSO/IPC.
- *Create adolescent-friendly services:* Ensure privacy, respectful communication, age-appropriate counseling, non-judgmental attitude and accessible services (contraception, STI screening, psychosocial support).
- *Ask sensitively about sexual history:* If an adolescent is sexually active or married, enquire in a structured, culturally sensitive manner: age of first activity, partner's age, consent, contraceptive use, STIs, psychosocial context.
- *Safeguarding protocols:* If you suspect sexual activity involving a minor below 18 years, or possible coercion/abuse, follow institutional child protection protocols. Document carefully.
- *Educate adolescents and families:* Use consultations to discuss anatomy, puberty, consent, safe sex, contraception, delaying first pregnancy, emotional readiness, healthy relationships, STIs and legal rights.
- *Advocate for sexual and reproductive rights:* Work with schools, NGOs, policy-makers to promote comprehensive sexuality education, awareness of the age of consent law, and the importance of delaying marriage, first birth and reducing adolescent pregnancy.
- *Be aware of cultural and regional variations:* In rural or under-resourced settings, child marriage and low contraceptive uptake are still prevalent—your role as an advocate, educator and clinician is crucial.

THE ONGOING DEBATE AND POTENTIAL POLICY DIRECTIONS

The age of consent remains a topic of debate in India. Some arguments and policy considerations:

- *Proposal to lower age to 16:* Some legal scholars and activists argue that because many adolescents are sexually active before 18, and the age of consent at 18 criminalizes consensual peer relationships, the threshold should be reconsidered.
- *Government's stance:* The Union Government has maintained that lowering the age from 18 would weaken child protection and create legal ambiguity.
- *Close-in-age exemption:* Introducing a "Romeo-and-Juliet" exception (whereby consensual sexual activity between adolescents close in age is de-criminalized) is being discussed to avoid the criminalization of adolescent peer sexual relationships.
- *Link with child marriage laws:* Age of consent interacts with the minimum age of marriage laws (female 18, male 21 under some proposals) and efforts to eliminate child marriage under the Prohibition of Child Marriage Act, 2006.
- *Aligning with global norms:* India's legal age of 18 aligns with the definition of a "child" under the United Nations Convention on the Rights of the Child (UNCRC) and India's commitments thereto.

From a policy perspective, the challenge is to strike a balance between *protecting minors* from sexual exploitation while also *respecting the emerging autonomy* of adolescents and ensuring that they can access sexual and reproductive health services without fear of criminalization or punitive repercussions.

Implications for Women's Health and Public Health

From the lens of gynecology and women's health, maintaining a clear and enforceable age of consent has several public-health benefits:

- *Prevention of early pregnancy:* Adolescents who engage in sexual activity early are at higher risk of unintended pregnancy, unsafe abortion, obstetric complications, low birth weight, maternal mortality, and poor neonatal outcomes. Legal thresholds help reinforce messages about delaying first birth and improving maternal health.
- *STI prevention:* Younger age of sexual initiation correlates with higher number of partners, lower contraceptive/condom use, and higher risk of STIs including HPV, which in turn raises risk of cervical cancer. Public health strategies must target adolescents with education, vaccination (e.g., HPV), screening and safe-sex counseling.

- *Empowerment and agency:* By clearly defining when consent is valid, we reinforce the need for healthy, consensual sexual relationships, respect for bodily autonomy and protection against coercion. This is integral to women's health and gender equality.
- *Reducing child marriage and its harms:* Child marriage is associated with early sexual debut, limited autonomy, interrupted education, increased obstetric risks and intergenerational poverty. Age of consent laws dovetail with efforts to eradicate child marriage and its negative health outcomes.
- *Health system readiness:* Healthcare providers must be trained in adolescent-friendly care, confidentiality, safeguarding protocols, legal frameworks and referral pathways. The intersection of law and medicine requires professional awareness to avoid harm and ensure rights are respected.

A NOTE OF CAUTION AND BALANCED PERSPECTIVE

While laws provide structure and protection, they are not sufficient alone. As gynecologists we must recognize:

- *Complex adolescence:* Adolescents are diverse in maturity, cognitive/emotional development, cultural background and risk exposure. Legal age is a threshold, but nuanced care is required.
- *Risk of victimizing adolescents:* Over-criminalization of consensual sexual activity among adolescents may drive behaviors underground, reduce trust in healthcare services and discourage open communication. We must advocate for balanced approaches.
- *Implementation gaps:* Many rural and marginalized communities may not be aware of the law or may still practice child marriage and early sexual debut. Legal safeguards must be matched by social change, education, empowerment and service access.
- *Clinical vs legal consent:* Medical consent (for treatment/procedure) and legal consent for sexual activity are distinct. Adolescents under 18 may consent to certain health services (depending on jurisdiction) but legally cannot consent to sex. Providers must be aware of both domains.
- *Holistic sexual education:* Laws cannot substitute for comprehensive sexuality education (CSE). Adolescents need accurate, age-appropriate information about sex, consent, relationships, contraception, STIs, power dynamics and respectful partnerships.

CONCLUSION

In India, the age of consent for sexual activity is firmly set at *18 years.* This legal standard serves as a protective measure for minors, aligns with adolescent health imperatives and signals societal commitment to sexual-health, rights and equity. For gynecologists, this means being aware of the legal context, delivering adolescent-friendly care, advocating for preventive and educational strategies, and supporting young people in making healthy choices.

At the same time, as India evolves demographically, socially and medically, the debate around age of consent and adolescent autonomy continues. We must engage with nuance, recognizing both the need for strong protection of minors and the importance of ensuring that adolescents can access the sexual and reproductive healthcare they need, when they need it.

In my practice, I encourage parents, educators and adolescents alike to view age of consent not only as a legal hurdle but as a springboard for conversation: about readiness, respect, responsibility and reproductive health. By doing so, we can help create a generation that is informed, empowered and healthy.

SUGGESTED READING

1. AgeOfConsent. (2025). The Age of Consent in India. [online] Available from https://www.ageofconsent.net/world/india [Last accessed January, 2026].
2. IJME. (2024). The Law Commission report on the age of consent: denying justice and autonomy to adolescents. [online] Available from https://ijme.in/articles/law-commission-of-india-report-on-the-age-of-consent-denying-justice-and-autonomy-to-adolescents/?galley=html [Last accessed January, 2026].
3. Lawbeat. (2025). Centre tells Supreme Court: No change in age of consent, 18 is non-negotiable. [online] Available from https://lawbeat.in/supreme-court-news-updates/centre-tells-supreme-court-no-change-in-age-of-consent-18-is-legally-non-negotiable-1514012 [Last accessed January, 2026].
4. NDTV: (2023). 10 Years to 18: The History of Age of Consent in India. [online] Available from https://www.ndtv.com/india-news/10-years-to-18-the-history-of-age-of-consent-in-india-4436742 [Last accessed January, 2026]
5. Pitre A, Lingam L. Age of consent: challenges and contradictions of sexual violence and law in India. Sex Reprod Health Matters. 2021;29(2):1878656.
6. Ribhu R. (2025) Understanding POCSO and why lowering the age of consent below 18 is dangerous. [online] Available from https://www.ndtv.com/opinion/understanding-posco-and-why-lowering-the-age-of-consent-below-18-is-dangerous-9106273 [Last accessed January, 2026].
7. Singh K. (2025). Rethinking the Age of Consent in India. [online] Available from https://www.theindiaforum.in/law/rethinking-age-consent-india [Last accessed January, 2026].
8. The Week. (2025). Age of consent around the world. [online] Available from https://theweek.com/92121/ages-of-consent-around-the-world [Last accessed January, 2026].

14 CHAPTER

Sensate Focus Therapy

Sujoy Dasgupta

INTRODUCTION

Sensate focus therapy is a prominent intervention for addressing sexual dysfunction in both men and women. Initially developed by Masters and Johnson, sensate focus therapy encourages individuals to explore and discover their own sensations, particularly genital sensations, often as a homework assignment after receiving therapist instructions. The core methodology involves a series of structured touching exercises designed to reduce performance anxiety and enhance tactile awareness, serving as both a diagnostic and therapeutic tool. This approach redirects attention from goal-oriented sexual performance to the nonjudgmental exploration of physical sensations, fostering a deeper appreciation for intimacy. Specifically, it helps individuals disengage from "spectatoring," a form of self-focused cognitive distraction that can impede sexual function by shifting focus from performance pressures to the present moment of sensory experience.

THE TECHNIQUE OF DETAILS

Sensate focus therapy, as a cornerstone of sex therapy, primarily involves structured exercises designed to re-sensitize individuals to nongenital touch and gradually progress to genital touch, thereby reducing performance pressure and fostering intimacy.

The core principle involves a "stop-start" method and other regulatory or "sexofunctional" techniques, including postural, respiratory, and motor exercises, which aim to habituate and desensitize individuals to arousal sensations and slow down psychophysiological and motor dynamics during excitement. Moreover, the integration of awareness-based methods, such as those described in Gestalt therapy, can further augment sensate focus techniques by promoting present-centeredness and fostering a continuum of awareness during sexual encounters. Indeed, the combined approach of behavioral techniques with pharmacotherapy often yields superior and more durable outcomes compared to monotherapy for various sexual dysfunctions, underscoring the benefits of holistic treatment strategies.

Detailed instruction about each step is given and the feedback is collected regarding the progress. Only if the progress is satisfactory, the couple will be guided to move to the next step. The stages of this assignment are based on the terminology used by Masters and Johnson and it includes nongenital sensate focus, genital sensate focus and vaginal containment.

Nongenital Sensate Focus

It improves the communication, awareness and intimacy among the couple by understanding each other's concerns. The partners are promoted to enjoy the physical contact but strict instruction should be given to abstain from sexual abstinence and from touching genitals and woman's breast. Men often achieve erection this time. However, they find it difficult to maintain and often they concentrate on the strength of erection and the girth and the length of the penis. They should be instructed to shift their focus from erection to pleasurable sensation.

Genital Sensate Focus

If a couple successfully went through the nongenital sensate focus, they should be instructed for genital sensate focus. Here they can enjoy genital contact to identify and focus on pleasurable sensation without having penetrative sex. Caressing partner's genitals using lubricants often heightens the arousal.

Vaginal Containment

This is very important stage because it involves vaginal penetration of penis, which often involves anxiety in individuals. When both are sexually comfortable, the woman should insert the man's penis into her vagina, preferably in woman-top or side-to-side position. The man has to lie still, focusing on any pleasurable genital sensation. It should be repeated up to three times in one occasion. If this stage is felt pleasurable by both, they can introduce the movement but the woman should start moving first.

The sensate focus therapy conforms to the PLISSIT model, described by Annon. It involves Permission giving (assuring the client that his thoughts or beliefs are not negatively affecting the partner), Limited Information (information about the particular sexual problem is given to the client), Specific Suggestion (sensate focus and homework assignment) and Intensive Sex therapy (insight oriented and psychosexual approach to make him aware of his feeling).

FEMALE SEXUAL DYSFUNCTION

This framework is particularly beneficial for treating female sexual dysfunction disorders, including female orgasmic disorder, female sexual interest/arousal disorder, and genito-pelvic pain/penetration disorder, which significantly impair women's quality of life. Holistic approaches that incorporate such behavioral therapies are increasingly utilized to promote sexual health and address these concerns effectively. Moreover, sensate focus therapy, often integrated with sex education and psychotherapy, has demonstrated efficacy in managing conditions such as penetration disorder, formerly known as vaginismus, by systematically desensitizing individuals to anxiety-provoking sexual encounters. This approach helps reframe sexual activity from a performance-oriented task to a mindful, sensory exploration, thereby reducing the cognitive and emotional barriers that contribute to sexual dysfunction. This is particularly relevant given that female sexual dysfunction is a prevalent condition that often lacks sufficient therapeutic options, with many women not seeking medical help for symptoms like reduced lubrication, pain during intercourse, and difficulties achieving orgasm. These psychological and interpersonal factors, often unaddressed in conventional treatments, underscore the necessity of comprehensive approaches that encompass behavioral strategies like sensate focus therapy, often complemented by psychoeducation and couples therapy.

MALE SEXUAL DYSFUNCTION

While mindfulness-based approaches have been extensively studied in women, their specific influence on male sexuality remains less explored, with current research suggesting potential benefits across various components of sexual activity. The application of mindfulness to male sexual health extends to mitigating psychological barriers to sexual satisfaction, such as self-consciousness and distraction during intimacy, thereby fostering a more embodied and present sexual experience. This integration of mindfulness within sensate focus therapy provides a robust framework for addressing the multifaceted nature of sexual dysfunction by re-establishing a connection between mind and body, thereby moving beyond the limitations of purely pharmacological interventions that often fail to address psychological components of sexual health. The cultivation of mindful awareness can effectively reframe experiences of sexual activity, fostering an increase in sexual self-efficacy and overall sexual functioning, as evidenced by significant improvements observed in clinical trials. Beyond its direct impact on sexual function, mindfulness has also been demonstrated to reduce psychological stress, anxiety, and depression, which are frequently co-occurring factors contributing to male sexual dysfunction.

For men with erectile dysfunction, a combined approach of pharmacological solutions with psychotherapy, including sensate focus therapy, has shown significant therapeutic value in improving sexual satisfaction and overall well-being beyond just erectile function. Furthermore, sensate focus techniques specifically help to alleviate performance anxiety by shifting the focus from erectile rigidity to mutual pleasure and sensory exploration, which can indirectly facilitate improved erectile responses.

Premature ejaculation can be effectively managed through behavioral techniques, including sensate focus therapy, which teach individuals to control and delay ejaculation by increasing awareness of arousal levels and implementing "stop-start" or squeeze techniques. These exercises, often facilitated through guided instructions, aim to enhance ejaculatory control by systematically desensitizing individuals to high levels of arousal, thereby prolonging sexual encounters and increasing satisfaction for both partners. Pharmacological interventions such as dapoxetine or topical anesthetics are frequently combined with these behavioral strategies to provide a comprehensive management approach for premature ejaculation, often yielding superior outcomes than either modality alone.

Male hypoactive sexual desire disorder, characterized by a persistent or recurrent deficiency or absence of sexual fantasies and desire for sexual activity, can be significantly ameliorated through sensate focus therapy by recalibrating the individual's focus from performance demands to the intrinsic pleasure of touch and intimacy. By de-emphasizing goal-oriented sexual activity, this approach can reduce pressure and enable a more organic rediscovery of sexual interest and responsiveness. This reorientation helps address the underlying psychological components of low desire, fostering a positive feedback loop where reduced anxiety leads to increased engagement and, consequently, a resurgence of sexual interest.

Delayed ejaculation, characterized by a persistent or recurrent difficulty, delay, or inability to achieve ejaculation despite adequate sexual stimulation, can also benefit from sensate focus therapy by addressing performance pressure and enhancing nongenital pleasure. However, there is lack of studies on role of sensate focus in delayed ejaculation.

KEY POINTS

- Sensate focus represents nonpharmacological treatment for almost all types of sexual dysfunctions in men and women
- It basically involves understanding own genital and nongenital sensation to reduce anxiety and improve sexual performances
- Combination of sensate focus and pharmacotherapy works better than monotherapy
- Sensate focus consists of nongenital sensate, genital sensate and vaginal containment
- Couples should be clearly instructed how to practice sensate focus

SUGGESTED READING

1. Adam F, Favez N, Pirard C, Wyns C, Equeter C, Grimm E, et al. Assessment of sexual function before medically assisted procreation: A mixed-methods study among a sample of infertile women and men cared for in a fertility center. Sex Reprod Healthcare. 2023;38:100922.

2. Ågmo A, Laan E. The Sexual Incentive Motivation Model and Its Clinical Applications. J Sex Res. 2023;60(7):969-88.
3. Annon JS. The Behavioral Treatment of Sexual Problems: Brief Therapy. New York: Harper & Row; 1976.
4. Avery-Clark C, Weiner L, Adams-Clark AA. Sensate Focus for Sexual Concerns: an Updated, Critical Literature Review. Curr Sexual Health Rep. 2019; 11(2):84.
5. Banbury S, Chandler C, Erridge S, Olvera J del R., Turner J, Lusher J. A Preliminary Study Looking at the Use of Mindful Compassion and Cannabis Suppositories for Anodyspareunia among Men Who Have Sex with Men (MSM). Psychoactives. 2024;3(3):384.
6. Brotto LA, Atallah S, Carvalho J, Gordon E, Pascoal PM, Reda M, et al. Psychological and interpersonal dimensions of sexual function and dysfunction: recommendations from the fifth international consultation on sexual medicine (ICSM 2024). Sex Med Rev. 2025;13(2):118-43.
7. Gewirtz-Meydan, A. Adapting Sensate Focus for Sexual Abuse Survivors: A Trauma-Informed Approach to Reclaiming Body and Intimacy. Sexual Health Compuls. 2025;32(3):205-20.
8. Gupta K, Patel AK. Mindfulness-based Therapy for management of Female Sexual Dysfunction and Psychological Well-being. In: Taukeni SG (Ed). Acceleration of the Biopsychosocial Model in Public Health. United States: IGI Global; 2022.
9. Kempeneers P. Revue systématique des essais consacrés aux traitements psycho-comportementaux de l'éjaculation prématurée. Sexologies. 2021;31(1):33.
10. Linschoten M, Weiner L, Avery-Clark C. Sensate focus: a critical literature review. Sexual Relation Ther. 2016;31(2):230.
11. Memik O, Voyvoda B, Ustuner M, Karsli O, Halat AO, Ozcan L. Regular penis-root masturbation: A promising behavioral treatment method for lifelong premature ejaculation. Prog Urol. 2023;33(15-16):1008-13.
12. Mestre-Bach G, Blycker GR, Potenza MN. Behavioral Therapies for Treating Female Sexual Dysfunctions: A State-of-the-Art Review. J Clin Med. 2022;11(10):2794.
13. Mosher DL. Awareness in gestalt sex therapy. J Sex Marit Ther. 1979;5(1):41.
14. Pastore AL, Fuschi A, Salhi YA, Velotti G, Capone L, Martoccia A., et al. Pelvic muscle floor rehabilitation as a therapeutic option in lifelong premature ejaculation: Long-term outcomes. Eur Urol Suppl. 2018;17(8):317.
15. Peixoto MM. Mindfulness, Self-Compassion, and Acceptance as Predictors of Sexual Satisfaction in Cisgender Heterosexual Men and Women. Healthcare. 2023;11(13):1839.
16. Quinta-Gomes AL, Janssen E, Adaikan G, Nobre P. Sexual Inhibition and Sexual Excitation Profiles in Men with and Without Erectile Disorder. Urology. 2021;161:71.
17. Ramanathan V, Redelman M. Sexual dysfunctions and sex therapy: The role of a general practitioner. Aust J Gen Pract. 2020;49(7):412.
18. Rodríguez MFV, Sánchez-Sánchez LC, García-Montes JM, Petisco C. A Scoping Review of the Influence of Mindfulness on Men's Sexual Activity. Int J Environment Res Public Health. 2023;20(4):3739.

19. Salonia A, Bettocchi C, Boeri L, Capogrosso P, Carvalho J, Çilesiz NC, et al. European Association of Urology Guidelines on Sexual and Reproductive Health—2021 Update: Male Sexual Dysfunction. Eur Urol. 2021;80(3):333.
20. Tang Y, Jing L, Liu Y, Wang H. Association of mindfulness on state-trait anxiety in choking-susceptible athletes: mediating roles of resilience and perceived stress. Front Psychol. 2023;14:1232929.
21. Vaishnav M, Saha G, Mukherji A, Vaishnav P. Principles of Marital Therapies and Behavior Therapy of Sexual Dysfunction. Indian J Psychiatry. 2020;62(Suppl 2):S213-S222.
22. Wiederman MW. Don't Look Now: The Role of Self-Focus in Sexual Dysfunction. Fam J. 2001;9(2):210.

15 CHAPTER

Cognitive Behavioral Sex Therapy

Vandana Rani Bhuriya

INTRODUCTION

The World Health Organization (WHO) defines sexual health as "a state of physical, emotional, mental and social well-being in relation to sexuality," with "the possibility of having pleasurable and safe sexual experiences, free of coercion, discrimination, and violence". Persistent difficulties experienced by a person or couple during any stage of normal sexual activity (desire, arousal, orgasm) or any pain during sexual intercourse is labelled as sexual dysfunction. Sexual dysfunction in either male or female can cause significant negative impact on the quality of life of the couple due to the underlying psychological distress and relationship problems. Thoughts, behavior and emotions are inter-connected, so, we need evidence-based framework to deal with these multi-dimensional issues. Cognitive behavior therapy (CBT) is a structured and goal-oriented form of psychotherapeutic treatment which provides a non-pharmacological approach towards treatment of sexual dysfunction. The main focus of CBT in sexual dysfunction is to address the negative thought patterns causing sexual dysfunction, improving communication and providing a supportive environment.

COGNITIVE BEHAVIORAL MODEL FOR SEXUAL DYSFUNCTION

Cognitive distortions and irrational behavior can lead to distress and sexual dysfunctions.

Cognitive Component

In reference to sexual health, cognition refers to beliefs and thoughts of persons towards themselves, their partners and sexuality. Cognitive distortions can be negative thoughts about body image, sexual performances and self-worth, etc. The examples of maladaptive cognitive thoughts in sexual dysfunctions are mentioned below:

- I must satisfy my partner each and every time.
- I am inadequate if I am not able to satisfy my partner.
- My body is unattractive and undesirable.
- Sex should always be perfect.

Due to such type of thoughts, mind is anxious and only self-focused which can deviate mental attention of any person away from arousal and orgasm. Over the time, there is a vicious circle of apprehension, frustration, failure, sexual dysfunction and escapism.

Behavioral Component

Avoiding sexual activity and physical intimacy, seeking extra-ordinary reassurance in the relationship and over-monitoring their performance comes in the behavior of some persons. According to their judgement, this can reduce their anxiety and embarrassment. However, such behavior can give them comfort for a short duration but is a cause for sexual dysfunction in long term.

Emotional and Physiological Interplay

Negative emotions like fear, guilt, shame and anxiety activates sympathetic nervous system which interferes with sexual arousal and performance. This further exacerbates the sexual dysfunction.

COGNITIVE BEHAVIORAL THERAPY (CBT) FOR SEXUAL DYSFUNCTION

CBT is short term psychotherapy mainly focused on symptoms. The main objective is to break maladaptive cognitive-affective-behavioral chains and replace these thoughts with reality-based cognitions. The interventions of CBT are structured around the following components:

- Identification of the problem and amendment of maladaptive sexual cognitive thoughts.
- Strategies to reduce performance anxiety.
- Improvement of communication and emotional intimacy.
- Development of practical and realistic expectations about sex.
- Restructuring of adaptive sexual behaviors and mindfulness to focus more on pleasure than performance.

Comprehensive assessment is the first step for finding reasons behind sexual troubles. This includes

- History-detailed sexual history including the onset of problem, duration of symptoms, level of psychological distress, relationship history with attention on partner's attitude, emotional intimacy and rapport with the partner. History of any chronic diseases and medications should also be ruled out.
- Psychological evaluation to rule out anxiety disorder, body image concerns and mood disorders.
- Cognitive assessment to diagnose any type of sexual opinions and maladaptive thoughts.

After detailed evaluation, the origin can be divided into cognitive, emotional, behavioral, relationship cause to understand the mechanism of dysfunction and formulate further strategies.

COGNITIVE STRATEGIES IN CBT FOR SEXUAL DYSFUNCTION

Cognitive Restructuring

This includes modification of maladaptive thoughts associated with emotional distress. Cognitive restructuring helps in identification of irrational and self-defeating beliefs and helps the individual in rephrasing these beliefs which can further reduce the stress associated with it. For example:

- *Irrational thought:* "If I can't maintain an erection, my partner will lose respect for me."
- *Rational alternative:* "Erection difficulties do not define my worth or masculinity and occasional erection difficulties are common."

Addressing Core Beliefs

CBT encourages clients to recognize the deep-seated schemas like guilt, shame and restrictive attitudes towards sexual activity and replace them with more positive, sex-affirming beliefs. Some Cultural beliefs are:

- "Good women don't enjoy sex."
- "It's wrong to express sexual desire"

Cognitive reframing—"Desire is a natural part of a loving relationship which should be enjoyed by every woman."

Rigid, self-critical beliefs have to be replaced by flexible, realistic, and self-accepting ones, which can further reduce anxiety and improve sexual functions.

Mindfulness-based Approaches

Mindfulness and acceptance techniques help the patients to shift the focus from performance to sensory experience. By implementing nonjudgmental awareness, clients can reduce self-monitoring and enhance pleasure.

BEHAVIORAL TECHNIQUES IN CBT FOR SEXUAL DYSFUNCTION

The behavioral interventions used in CBT are:

- *Sensate focus:* It is the psychosexual skill exercise in which couples engage in structured, non-demand touching exercises designed to decrease performance pressure and rebuild physical intimacy. The focus gradually shifts from non-genital to genital stimulation and eventually to coitus as comfort increases. The counsellor's role is to highlight the sexual exchange, with a focus on pleasure rather than on intercourse performance.

- *Exposure therapy:* Exposure techniques provide graded exposure to the feared situations like fear of penetration or sexual initiation. This step wise exposure and confrontation of feared situations lead to desensitization and further reduces anxiety of the individual.
- *Behavioral experiments:* Real life experiments are conducted to see the actual outcome of the beliefs of an individual. For example: a client who fears rejection after discussing sexual difficulties with a partner can be guided to communicate openly and observe the actual outcome.
- *Communication and relationship skills:* Improving verbal and non-verbal communication in a relationship is an important component of CBT. Resolution of conflicts and emotional expression in a relationship enhances intimacy and mutual understanding which are important for sexual satisfaction.
- *Relaxation training:* Relaxation tools like deep breathing exercises, pelvic muscle management, and progressive muscle relaxation are introduced in CBT to promote comfort and relaxation as it is perceived as foundational for pleasure and arousal. Deep breathing exercises can be done during couple spooning and it provides comfort, relaxation and warmth. Breath matching during cuddling also promotes comfort and co-operation in a relationship. Progressive muscle relaxation involves tightening muscles, holding and appreciating the tension, releasing the tension, and then, enjoying the sensation of relaxation.

APPLICATIONS OF CBT TO SPECIFIC SEXUAL DYSFUNCTIONS

The aims, components and effects of CBT in different types of sexual dysfunction are specified in **Table 1**.

Role of Partner in CBT

Partner involvement in CBT enhances communication and shared responsibility in the treatment of any sexual disorder. This further supports behavioral exercises and boost relationship dynamics resulting in better gratification rates.

Advantages of CBT

- Both relationship and psychological dimensions are addressed
- Long-term changes can be developed through skill development
- Evidence-based tool

Disadvantages of CBT

- Less effective for dysfunctions due to organic causes
- Less availability of trained professionals for CBT
- Requires constant active participation and motivation

TABLE 1: Applications of CBT in sexual dysfunctions.

Sexual dysfunction	*Aims of CBT*	*Components of CBT*	*Effects of CBT*
Female orgasmic disorder (FOD)	• To promote changes in thoughts • To decrease anxiety • To increase orgasmic ability and sexual satisfaction	• Sex education • Cognitive restructuring • Systematic desensitization • Sensate focus • Communication training • Kegel exercises • Directed masturbation	Increased chances of achieving orgasm through masturbation or coitus
Female sexual interest/arousal disorder	• To promote motivation for engaging in sexual relationships • To improve couple's relationship and skills of erotic stimulation	All components in FOD plus: • Sexual fantasy training • Orgasm consistency training	Improvements in cognitive, behavioral, and marital functioning with greater sexual satisfaction
Genito-pelvic pain/penetration disorder (vaginismus)	• To focus on pain, reduce fear of pain and achieve pain control in sexual contexts • To (re)establish satisfying sexual functioning • To reduce muscle contraction in the pelvic floor and promote lubrication during sexual intercourse	All components in FOD plus: • Progressive muscle relaxation • Abdominal breathing • Vaginal dilatation • Distraction techniques including focusing on sexual imagery • Rehearsal of coping self-statements	• Reduced fear of coitus and avoidance behavior Reduced negative penetration beliefs • Reduced dyspareunia and improved sexual function
Erectile Dysfunction (ED)	To reduce fear of performance anxiety, catastrophic thinking, and avoidance	• Behavioral interventions • Sensate focus and graded exposure • Sex education • Cognitive restructuring	Reduced fear of failure and improved outcomes
Premature ejaculation	• To reduce anxiety and increasing control • To recognize early signs of arousal and delay ejaculation	• The "start-stop" or "squeeze" method • Relaxation and mindfulness techniques	Decreased anxiety about sexual adequacy

CONCLUSION

Cognitive behavioral therapy is an indispensable tool in modern sexual medicine which addresses the interplay between thought, behavior and emotions. It provides a structured evidence-based framework for management of sexual dysfunctions. Both cognitive and behavioral strategies in CBT help achieve sexual gratification, intimacy in relationship and a healthy sexual life.

KEY POINTS

- CBT is a structured goal-oriented form of non-pharmacological psychotherapy for sexual dysfunction.
- CBT deals with the interplay of cognitive factors, behavioral factors and emotional factors causing sexual dysfunction.
- Comprehensive evaluation and formulation of the cause is the cornerstone of CBT.
- Cognitive restructuring, addressing core beliefs and mindfulness and acceptance techniques are cognitive strategies of CBT.
- Behavioral strategies include sensate focus, exposure therapy, behavior experiments, communication skills and relationship training.
- Involvement of partner in CBT enhances better outcomes and improves intimate relationship.
- CBT offers promising results in the management of sexual dysfunction due to non-organic causes.

SUGGESTED READING

1. Beck JS. Cognitive behavior therapy: Basics and beyond, 2nd edition. New York: Guilford Press; 2011.
2. Brotto LA, Luria M. Mindfulness-based sex therapy for women with sexual interest/arousal disorder. Mindfulness. 2014;5(1):1-12.
3. Hong A, Ri-Hui, H, Yun-Rong, Z, Ran T. Cognitive-Behavioral Therapy. In: Xiaochu, Z, Jie S, Ran T (Eds). Substance and Non-Substance Addiction. Advances in Experimental Medicine and Biology. Springer: Singapore, 2017.
4. McCarthy BW, Wald LM. Cognitive-behavioral strategies and couples therapy in sexual dysfunction treatment. J Sex Marit Ther. 2013;39(3):193-210.
5. Mestre-Bach G, Blycker GR, Potenza, MN. Behavioral Therapies for Treating Female Sexual Dysfunctions: A State-of-the-Art Review. J Clin Med. 2022;11:2794.
6. Metz ME, Epstein N, Mccarthy B. Cognitive-behavioral therapy for sexual dysfunction. Philadelphia: Taylor & Francis; 2018.
7. Nobre PJ, Pinto-Gouveia J. Cognitive schemas associated with negative sexual experiences: Testing a model of cognitive-behavioral therapy for sexual dysfunctions. J Sex Res. 2008;45(4):372-81.
8. World Health Organization. Defining Sexual Health: Report of a Technical Consultation on Sexual Health, 28–31 January 2002. Geneva, Switzerland: World Health Organization; 2006.

16 CHAPTER

Sexual and Reproductive Rights

Madhu Kiran

INTRODUCTION

Reproductive behavior in humans is the reflection of various psychological, biological, social, cultural and interpersonal relationships. We have to understand that complexity of male/female psychology, societal norms and community ideologies play a significant role in our understanding of Reproductive health. By default women bear the adverse effects of reproductive health issues and their vulnerability, for obvious reasons, is increased due to biological, cultural, social and economic factors mostly working against them. Challenges often start in childhood and adolescents like—Malnourishment/ anemia, psychosexual trauma, Unwanted pregnancies, ST1, Sexual abuse and rape. In child bearing females there are other challenges like—Number of pregnancies, spacing between pregnancies due to limited choice of contraceptives and information about the complications of pregnancies, Unwanted pregnancy and unsafe abortion practices. Meeting Family planning needs are an important part of healthcare services but are usually difficult to achieve because of lack of information, limited choice of contraceptive methods and concerns about safety and side effects of these methods, poor access to quality healthcare services and family and partner's disapproval.

HOW BIG IS THE PROBLEM?

The World health organization (WHO) estimates that:

- About 123 million women worldwide especially in developing countries are not able to use contraceptive methods of their choice even if they want to.
- Only 57% of women (15–49 years) make informed decisions on sexual relations, contraception use and reproductive health care.
- A woman dies every two minutes due to pregnancy or childbirth complications.
- Among the 1.9 billion women of reproductive age(15–49 years), only 270 million can access contraception.
- Approximately 73 million induced abortions take place each year, and half of them are unsafe
- Almost one in three women, across their lifetime have been subjected to physical or sexual violence by an intimate partner or sexual violence by a non-partner

- Over one million sexually transmitted infections are acquired everyday
- Almost 500 million girls and women lack access to services and products for managing their menstruation with comfort and dignity.

HISTORY OF SEXUAL AND REPRODUCTIVE RIGHTS

Government—run Family planning programs have been running since early 1950, However population control leading to development and economic growth was always the main driving force.

In 1994, the International Conference on Population and Development (ICPD) in Cairo, Egypt birth of modern SRHR movement took place by bringing a paradigm shift in our understanding regarding Reproductive health. A Program of Action (PoA) was developed and was approved and adopted by 179 countries. In the PoA it was affirmed that sexual and reproductive health are universal human rights. It outlined global goals and objectives of improving reproductive health. These goals were based around central themes of free choice, women's empowerment and viewing sexual and reproductive health in terms of physical and emotional wellbeing.

Reproductive and sexual rights include human rights that are already recognized in National laws and in the Universal Declaration on Human Rights.

- Information, education, skills, support and services needed to make responsible decisions about sexuality consistent with their own values (sexuality)
- Bodily integrity and voluntary sexual relationships
- Full range of voluntary and accessible sexual and reproductive health services
- Express one's sexual orientation without violence or discrimination.
- Decide freely and responsibly the number, spacing and timing of their children and the information and means to do so.
- Attain the highest standard of sexual and reproductive health.
- Make decision concerning reproduction free of discrimination, coercion or violence.

In 1997, the World Congress of Sexology (WAS) issued the Valencia Declaration of Sexual Rights. In March 2014, these Rights were revised and expanded to include 16 sexual rights.

1. The right to equality and non-discrimination.
2. The right to life, liberty, and security of the person
3. The right to autonomy and bodily integrity
4. The right to be free from torture and cruel, inhuman, or degrading treatment or punishment.
5. The right to be free from all forms of violence and coercion.
6. The right to privacy

7. The right to the highest attainable standard of health, including sexual health; with the possibility of pleasurable, satisfying, and safe sexual experiences
8. The right to enjoy the benefits of scientific progress and its application
9. The right to information
10. The right to education and the right to comprehensive sexuality education
11. The right to enter, form, and dissolve marriage and similar types of relationships based on equality and full and free consent
12. The right to decide whether to have children, the number and spacing of children, and to have the information and the means to do so
13. The right to the freedom of thought, opinion, and expression
14. The right to the freedom of association and peaceful assembly
15. The right to participation in public and political life
16. The right to access to justice, remedies, and redress (6)

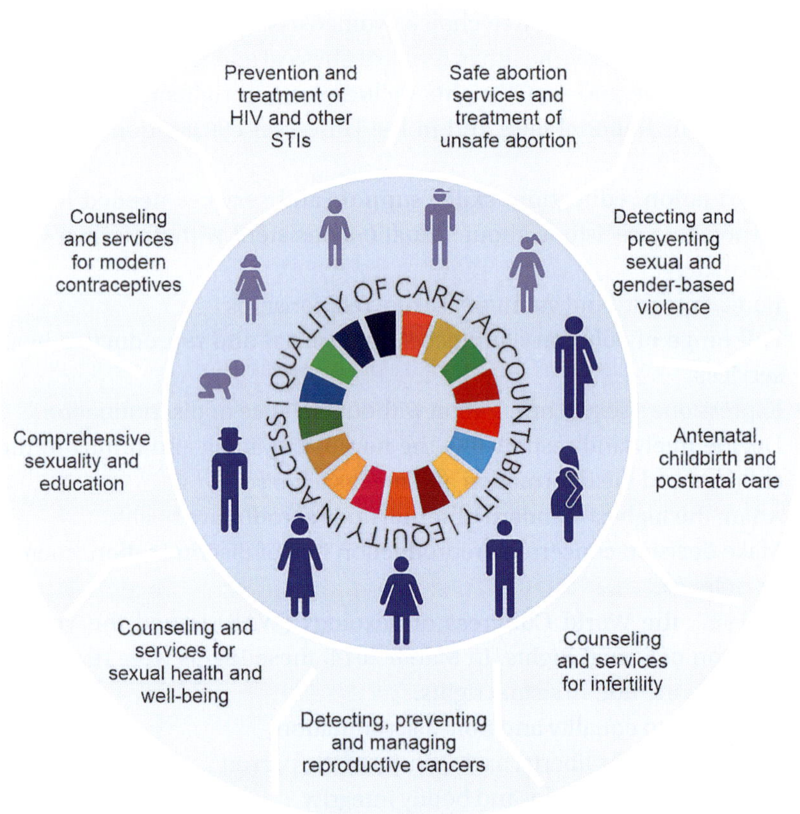

Fig. 1: A comprehensive definition of sexual and reproductive health and rights. *Source:* UNFPA. (2019). SRHR-An Essential Element of Universal Health. [online] Available from https://www.unfpa.org/publications/sexual-and-reproductive-health-and-rights-essential-element-universal-health-coverage [Last accessed January, 2026].

TABLE 1: Overview of scope of rights of sexual and reproductive health.

Sexual health and rights	*Reproductive health and rights*
Primary focus • Sexuality • Identity • Personal relationships beyond reproduction	*Primary focus* • The reproductive processes, functions and systems through all stages of life
Scope of rights • The right to define your own sexuality, gender identity and gender expression • The right to choose whether and when to be sexually active, as well as who to choose as a sexual partner • The right to have safe, consensual and pleasurable sexual experiences, free from violence, coercion and discrimination • The right to comprehensive sexuality education	*Scope of rights* • The right to decide freely and responsibly the number and spacing and timing of children • The right to access and be informed about contraception and family planning • The right to access quality maternal healthcare, including services for pregnancy, childbirth and postnatal care • The right to safe and legal abortion services as permitted by law

SEXUAL AND REPRODUCTIVE HEALTH AND RIGHTS

Sexual and reproductive health and rights are two distinct yet interconnected concepts that are essential for overall wellbeing. WHO defined Sexual Health as the state of physical mental and social wellbeing in relation to sexuality. It requires a positive and respectful approach to sexuality and sexual relationships as well as the possibility of having pleasurable and safe sexual experiences, free of coercion discrimination and violence. Reproductive health is defined in ICPD as a state of complete physical, mental and social wellbeing in all matters relating to the reproductive health system and to its functions and processes. It implies that people have the capability to reproduce and the freedom to decide if when and how often to do so **(Table 1)**.

VIOLATIONS OF SEXUAL AND REPRODUCTIVE HEALTH RIGHTS

Despite obligations and declarations, the neglect of these rights remains pervasive, most often not due to a lack of resources but to the widespread disregard for women's human rights including their dignity, bodily integrity and autonomy.

Violations of sexual and reproductive health and rights are mainly due to deeply ingrained beliefs and societal values pertaining to women's sexuality. Patriarchal constructs of women's role within the family and society at large perpetuate harmful expectations regarding women's primary role as child bearers and care givers, resulting in failure to sufficiently prioritize women's rights, in particular their sexual and reproductive health.

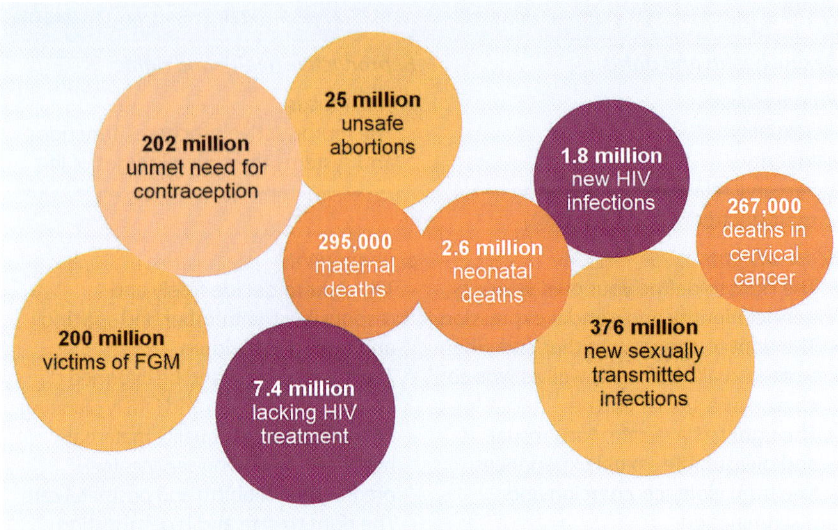

Fig. 2: The unfinished agenda.
Source: Government of Kenya, Government of Denmark, UNFPA Nairobi, Kenya. (2019). ICPD Nairobi Summit 2025. [online] Available from https://iawg.net/events/nairobi-summit-icpd25 [Last accessed January, 2026].

Restrictions on, or lack of access to sexual and reproductive healthcare, in particular contraception, emergency contraception, prophylactic treatment or comprehensive abortion care can cause a range of human rights violations and irreversible harm, child/early marriage and adolescent pregnancy, or repeated pregnancies without adequate spacing have a devastating impact on women's health and sometimes fatal consequences. Vulnerability of women to sexual and gender based violence (GBV) includes variety of abuses, sexual threats and coercion, exploitation, molestation, humiliation, incest, trafficking smuggling, forced marriage, and forced prostitution.

THE WAY FORWARD

States have obligations to respect, protect and fulfill rights related to sexual and reproductive health. To fulfill these obligations states must repeal or eliminate laws, practices and policies that criminalize, obstruct or undermine access by individuals or a particular group to a sexual or reproductive health facilities services, goods and information. There should be comprehensive inclusion of SRHR in the context of UHC, analyze SRHR needs of the population and mobilize all key stakeholders for implementing interventions. States should also analyze supply and demand side requirements and prioritize interventions based on people's needs. It is important to integrate SRHR services in health centers and hospitals, health benefit packages in national health policies.

There should be political commitment to mobilizing and coordinating funds to implement evidence driven actions for better management of improving overall maternal health, unwanted pregnancies, access to safe and legal abortion.

STRATEGIC ACTIONS THAT CAN BE TAKEN BY NGOS AND OTHER FORUMS

1. Support family planning and birth spacing services by advocating and lobbying to create funds
2. Reproductive health services for men, women and adolescents should be promoted through information, education and other forms of communication

Table 1	Key SRHR and UHC targets in the SDGs
3.1	By 2030, **reduce the global maternal mortality ratio** to less than 70 per 100,000 live births
3.2	By 2030, **end preventable deaths of newborns and children under 5 years of age,** with all countries aiming to reduce neonatal mortality to at least as low as 12 per 1,000 live births and under-5 mortality to at least as low as 25 per 1,000 live births
3.3	By 2030, **end the epidemics of AIDS**, tuberculosis, malaria and neglected tropical diseases and combat hepatitis, water-borne diseases and other communicable diseases
3.7	By 2030, **ensure universal access to sexual and reproductive health-care services,** including for family planning, information and education, and the integration of reproductive health into national strategies and programmes
3.8	**Achieve universal health coverage**, including financial risk protection, access to quality essential health-care services and access to safe, effective, quality and affordable essential medicines and vaccines for all
5.2	**Eliminate all forms of violence against all women and girls** in the public and private spheres, including trafficking and sexual and other types of exploitation
5.3	**Eliminate all harmful practices**, such as child, early and forced marriage and female genital mutilation
5.6	Ensure **universal access to sexual and reproductive health and reproductive rights** as agreed in accordance with the Programme of Action of the International Conference on Population and Development and the Beijing Platform for Action and the outcome documents of their review conferences
	Unlike the MDGs, the SDGs explicitly recognize sexual and reproductive health as being essential to health, development and women's empowerment

Fig. 3: Key SRHR and UHC targets in the SDGs.
Courtesy: United Nations SDGs

3. Safe contraception methods and family planning services should be taught to both males and females alike
4. Impact of Gender Based Violence (GBV) on women can be reduced by campaigns which also include young boys and girls in these activities.

Sexual and Reproductive Health and Rights in INDIA

Medical Termination of Pregnancy Act, Prohibition of Child Marriage Act, Maternity Benefit Act and various Supreme Court rulings to insure dignity in sterilization and abortions beyond 20 weeks in special cases are some of the core components of SRHR in India, but the real challenges are in Adolescent health due to lack of information, Health disparities in access to care based on socio-economic factors and Challenges in ensuring consistent access to quality reproductive health care services.

KEY POINTS

Sexual and reproductive health are integral elements of the right of everyone, to the enjoyment of the highest attainable standards of physical and mental health. Comprehensive SRH services include antenatal care, labor and child birth, postnatal care, and services for contraception and family planning, infertility, sexual health, intimate partner and sexual violence, abortion, STIs, and comprehensive sexuality education. Advancing universal SRH coverage requires a combination of political commitment and well defined and coherent strategies.

SUGGESTED READING

1. Annual report on UNFPA 2019 Unfinished Business- The pursuit of Rights and Choices for All.
2. Department of Economic and Social Affairs ICPD 94 Series Population and Development PoA adopted at International Conference on Population and Development Cairo Sept; 1994.
3. Glasier A, Gulnezoglu AM, Schmid GP, Moreno CG, Van look PF. Sexual and reproductive health: a matter of life and death. Lancet. 2006;368(9547):1595-607.
4. Leebetter R (1984). Thirty years of family planning in India. ASIAN Surv. 1984;24(7):736-58.
5. Nairobi Statement on ICPD 25 Sexual and Reproductive Health and Rights: an essential element in Universal Health Coverage.
6. OHCHR and Women's right and gender equality-Information series on sexual and reproductive health and rights 1996-2025.
7. Political declaration of high-level meeting on Universal Health Coverage: Resolution/Adopted by the general assembly; 2023.
8. Ross JA, Winfrey WL. Winfrey Unmet needs for contraception in the developing world and the former Soviet Union: An updated estimate in International family planning perspective. Int Fam Plan Perspect. 2002;28(3):138-43.
9. WAS. (2025). Declaration of sexual rights. [online] Available from: https://www.worldsexualhealth.net/_files/ugd/793f03_779f193815894895b9d1480bde676c37.pdf?index=true [Last accessed January, 2026].
10. WHO. (2023). Investing in sexual and reproductive health and rights; essential elements of universal health coverage. Geneva: WHO; 2023.
11. WHO South-East Asia /Health Topics/Reproductive Health July; 2025.

17 CHAPTER

Mindfulness-based Therapy for Management of Female Sexual Dysfunction

Shama Sultana

INTRODUCTION

Female Sexual Dysfunction (FSD) affects quality of life and relationships and is Defined as disturbances in sexual desire, arousal, orgasm, or pain:

- It Causes significant distress and interpersonal difficulties
- Mental health impairment is a major risk factor
- It is Characterized by Impaired sexual desire, arousal, or orgasm, Difficulty initiating or completing sexual activity, persistent or recurrent difficulties with orgasm Personal suffering and distress. Its key aspects are, Sexual response cycle: desire, arousal, orgasm
- *Arousal response:* vasocongestion, vaginal lubrication, genital swelling
- *Orgasmic disorders:* difficulty or absence of orgasm despite sufficient stimulation.

SEXUAL PAIN DISORDERS IN FEMALES

- *Dyspareunia:* Persistent genital pain during intercourse
- *Vaginismus:* Involuntary vaginal spasm interfering with penetration
- *Noncoital sexual pain disorder:* Genital pain induced by noncoital sexual stimulation, it may impact
- Distressing due to hectic lifestyles
- Significant impact on mental health and Quality of Life.

DIAGNOSING FEMALE SEXUAL DYSFUNCTION

- Symptoms must persist for ≥6 months
- Experienced in ≥75% of sexual encounters
- Causes clinically significant distress
- Approximately half of women report impaired sexual desire, arousal, or orgasm: Sexual health linked more strongly to mental health than physical function or age (especially in older women).

BACKGROUND

Sexual dysfunction is a clinically significant disturbance in an individual's ability to respond sexually, causing distress or impairment. According to DSM-5 criteria, it's characterized by a pattern associated with distress/

disability, influenced by individual vulnerability factors such as biological, psychological, and relational aspects. These factors contribute to the development of sexual dysfunction, impacting overall well-being.

PSYCHOLOGICAL RISK FACTORS FOR FEMALE SEXUAL DYSFUNCTION

Factors associated with female sexual dysfunction can be attributed to certain individual factors that could influence sexual response difficulties in females.

- *Individual vulnerability factors:* According to DSM-5, sexual dysfunction is a clinically significant issue that affects an individual's sexual response, causing notable distress or impairment in their daily life. It's marked by specific patterns that can be behavioral or psychological in nature.
- *Motivation:* The Incentive Motivation model suggests that sexual desire arises from engaging in sexual activity, rather than being a precursor. In contrast, Basson's model proposes that women are often in a state of sexual neutrality, and a range of motivating factors can trigger their desire, highlighting the complex link between motivation and sexual desire. Research supports this, identifying numerous reasons that motivate women's sexual desire.
- *Childhood sexual and emotional abuse:* Women survivors of child sexual abuse often experience low sexual desire, negative self-perceptions, anxiety, and depression. They tend to associate sex with negative emotions and exhibit lower genital arousal. However, research suggests that mindfulness-based interventions can be effective in addressing these issues, particularly for women with a history of child sexual abuse.
- *Body Image:* Research by Weiderman found that many young women experience body image self-consciousness during intimacy, which is linked to lower sexual self-esteem. This self-consciousness can lead to sexual avoidance, reduced assertiveness, and fewer sexual experiences. Additionally, another study suggests that self-focus can impact sexuality differently depending on whether a woman is sexually aroused or not.
- *Performance Anxiety and Negative Expectations:* Sexual dysfunction in females is often linked to performance anxiety, particularly fear of not meeting partner expectations or excessive need to please. This anxiety can inhibit physiological arousal, leading to sexual difficulties. Negative expectations also play a significant role, with research suggesting that women with negative sexual schemas are more likely to develop sexual dysfunctions. According to Barlow's model, individuals with sexual dysfunction often expect poor outcomes, feeling unable to change the course of events, which can impair sexual function.

PSYCHOLOGICAL THERAPIES AVAILABLE FOR FEMALE SEXUAL DYSFUNCTION

For decades, psychological treatments for female sexual dysfunction have built upon the behavioral techniques introduced by Masters and Johnson in 1970. Their approach, particularly "sensate focus exercises," remains a cornerstone of sex therapy, widely used by clinicians today.

- *Cognitive Behavioral Therapy (CBT):* Sensate focus exercises have been a primary treatment for low sexual desire and arousal in women, endorsed by the 2015 International Consultation on Sexual Medicine. However, further research is needed due to limited studies. Cognitive Behavioral Therapy offers an alternative approach, helping women challenge negative thoughts, learn relaxation techniques, and overcome avoidance behaviors to improve sexual function.
- Cognitive Behavioral Therapy has been shown to be effective in treating low sexual desire and arousal in women, with significant benefits for sexual satisfaction. Involving male partners in treatment can enhance outcomes. CBT also shows promise for addressing sexual pain, although more research is needed to establish guidelines. By targeting negative thought patterns and emotions, CBT can help women modulate their physical responses and improve their sexual experiences. Additionally, understanding the brain's role in pain perception can help women recognize the impact of thoughts and emotions on their physical sensations.
- *MBCT* (Mindfulness-based Cognitive therapies): Mindfulness-based therapies are increasingly being used in Western medicine to treat various conditions, including depression, anxiety, and chronic pain. These therapies help individuals develop skills such as acceptance, non-judgment, and non-reaction, allowing them to focus on the present moment and reduce cognitive distractions. Research has shown that mindfulness-based interventions can be effective in improving sexual function in women with low desire and arousal, reducing avoidance of sexual interaction, and alleviating sexual pain. Studies have also found that meditation can alter brain morphology and reduce pain intensity by changing brain activity patterns.
- *Mindfulness based Therapy:* Mindfulness is a conscious state of acceptance and present-moment awareness without judgment. Rooted in Buddhist Vipassana meditation, mindfulness-based therapies focus on cultivating acceptance, curiosity, and openness to experiences, allowing negative emotions to pass without attempting to change them. This approach differs from traditional cognitive-behavioral therapy in its emphasis on refined attention training, rather than cognitive restructuring or mood monitoring.

Sensate focus and mindfulness meditation share similarities in their focus on present-moment sensations and reduced self-monitoring. However, they differ in key ways: mindfulness can be practiced individually, making it accessible to those without partners or with anxiety issues, whereas sensate focus requires a partner. Additionally, mindfulness encompasses a broader range of attention targets, including breath, body sensations, and thoughts, whereas sensate focus primarily focuses on partner touch sensations.

Mindfulness can help individuals in several ways:

- By focusing on the present moment, it reduces worries about future outcomes during sexual activity.
- The non-striving aspect of mindfulness encourages letting go of expectations and goals, promoting a more accepting attitude.
- Nonjudgmental acceptance allows individuals to appreciate their current experience, even if it doesn't meet their desired level of sexual function, reducing the pressure to perform and promoting a more positive experience.

CHALLENGES AND ISSUES IN FEMALE SEXUAL DYSFUNCTION

- *Prevalence:* 10% of women experience distressing sexual dysfunction, while 20% report less disturbing sexual problems.
- *Common symptoms:* Low desire, low subjective arousal, and infrequent or absent orgasm.
- *Age and menopause:* Desire decreases with age and menopause, with greater distress after surgical menopause.
- *Limited understanding:* Need to better understand mechanisms of treatment effectiveness, particularly for psychological interventions like mindfulness.
- *Lack of approved treatments:* No USFDA-approved medications for female sexual dysfunction due to complex psychosocial and interpersonal factors.
- *Clinician discomfort:* Many clinicians feel uncomfortable discussing sexuality with patients and may underestimate its importance.

SOLUTIONS AND RECOMMENDATIONS

Online Mindfulness-based Therapies

Benefits:

- *Convenience and Privacy*:* Online therapies offer flexibility and anonymity, making it easier for women to seek help without feeling uncomfortable or embarrassed.
- **Community Support*:* Online platforms can connect women with similar experiences, providing a sense of community and support.

- *Improved Accessibility*: Online therapies can reach women in remote or underserved areas, bridging the gap in healthcare access.

Effectiveness:
- Studies have shown that online mindfulness-based cognitive behavioral therapy can significantly improve sexual desire, arousal, lubrication, orgasm, and overall sexual satisfaction in women.
- Mindfulness-based interventions have also been effective in reducing sexual distress, depression, and anxiety in women.
- Online CBT programs with mindfulness training have demonstrated promising results, with improvements sustained at follow-up assessments.

KEY COMPONENTS OF ONLINE MINDFULNESS-BASED THERAPIES

- *Mindfulness Training:* Focuses on developing present-moment awareness, reducing judgment, and increasing self-acceptance.
- *Psychoeducation:* Provides knowledge about sexual response, healthy relationships, and communication skills.
- *Sensate Focus:* A technique that helps women focus on physical sensations, building intimacy and pleasure.
- *Communication Exercises:* Enhances relationship communication and conflict resolution skills.

FUTURE DIRECTIONS

- Further research is needed to explore the long-term effects of online mindfulness-based therapies for female sexual dysfunction.
- Developing standardized online therapy programs and assessing their effectiveness in diverse populations is crucial.

TAKE HOME MESSAGE

Mindfulness-based therapies show promise in addressing female sexual dysfunction. Here's a summary of the benefits and key points:

Benefits of mindfulness-based therapies:
- Increased present-moment awareness: reduces distraction and increases attention to sexual experiences, promoting healthy sexual response
- Reduced negative sexual schemas: helps women overcome negative thoughts and emotions associated with sex
- Improved inter-relational context: enhances relationship communication and intimacy- Reduced symptoms of depression and anxiety: mindfulness-based cognitive therapies have been shown to decrease symptoms of depression and anxiety in women

Key findings:
- Mindfulness-based cognitive therapies have been effective in improving sexual function, reducing sexual distress, and alleviating symptoms of depression in women

- Studies have reported significant improvements in sexual desire, arousal, lubrication, orgasm, and overall sexual satisfaction
- Mindfulness-based interventions have been found to be feasible and effective in various formats, including online and group-based sessions

FUTURE RESEARCH DIRECTIONS

- *Mechanisms of action:* Further research is needed to understand how mindfulness-based therapies work and their potential benefits for female sexual dysfunction
- *Standardized treatment programs:* Developing standardized online therapy programs and assessing their effectiveness in diverse populations is crucial
- *Long-term effects:* Investigating the long-term benefits and potential risks of mindfulness-based therapies for female sexual dysfunction.

SUGGESTED READING

1. Andersson E, Walén C, Hallberg J, Paxling B, Dahlin M, Almlöv J, et al. (2011). A Randomized Controlled Trial of Guided Internet-delivered.
2. Andersson G. (2015). Internet-delivered psychological treatments. Annu Rev Clin Psychol. 2016:12:157-79.
3. Barlow DH. Causes of sexual dysfunction: the role of anxiety and cognitive interference. J Consult Clin Psychol. 1986;54(2):140-8.
4. Basson R, Gilks T. Women's sexual dysfunction associated with psychiatric disorders and their treatment. Women's Health (London, England), 2018;14:1745506518762664.
5. Bavelas JB, Coates L, Johnson T. Listeners as co-narrators. Journal of Personality and Social Psychology, 2000;79(6):941-52.
6. Beck AT, Beamesderfer A. Assessment of depression: the depression inventory. Mod Probl Pharmacopsychiatry. 1974;7(0):151-69.
7. Bishop SR, Lau M, Shapiro S, Carlson L, Anderson ND, Carmody J, et al. Mindfulness: A proposed operational definition. Clin Psychol: Sci Prac. 2004;11(3):230-41.
8. Brotto L, Atallah S, Johnson-Agbakwu C, Rosenbaum T, Abdo C, Byers E, et al. Psychological and interpersonal dimensions of sexual function and dysfunction. J Sex Med. 2016;13(4):538-71.
9. Brotto LA, Basson R, Carlson M, Zhu C. Impact of an integrated mindfulness and cognitive behavioural treatment for provoked vestibulodynia (IMPROVED): A qualitative study. Sex Relation Ther. 2013;28(1-2):3-19.
10. Brotto LA, Basson R, Smith KB, Driscoll M, Sadownik LA. (2013).
11. Brotto LA, Basson, R. Group mindfulness-based therapy significantly improves sexual desire in women. Behav Res Ther. 2014;57:43-54.
12. Brotto LA, Chivers ML, Millman R. Mindfulness improves genital subjective arousal concordance in women with sexual difficulties. 2013.
13. Brotto LA, Erskine Y, Carey M, Ehlen T, Finlayson S, Heywood M, et al. A brief mindfulness-based cognitive behavioral intervention improves sexual

functioning versus wait-list control in women treated for gynaecologic cancer. Gynecol Oncol. 2012;125(2):320-5.
14. Brotto LA, Seal BN, Rellini A. Pilot study of a brief cognitive behavioral versus mindfulness-based intervention for women with sexual distress and a history of childhood sexual abuse. J Sex Marit Ther. 2012;38(1):1-27.
15. Brotto LA, Yule M. Asexuality: Sexual orientation, paraphilia, sexual dysfunction, or none of the above? Arch Sex Behav. 2017;46(3):619-27.
16. Brotto LA. Mindful sex. Canadian J Hum Sex. 2013;22(2):63-8.
17. Cognitive Behavioral Therapy for Erectile Dysfunction. J Sex Med. 2011;8(10):2800-9.
18. de Jong D. The role of attention in sexual arousal: implications for treatment of sexual dysfunction. J Sex Res. 2009;46(2):237-48.
19. Dennerstein L, Guthrie JR, Hayes RD, DeRogatis LR, Lehert P. Sexual function, dysfunction, and sexual distress in a prospective, population-based sample of mid-aged, Australian-born women. J Sex Med. 2008;5(10):2291-9.
20. Doss BD, Thum YM, Sevier M, Atkins DC, Christensen A. Improving relationships: Mechanisms of change in couple therapy. J Consult Clin Psychol. 2005;73(4):624-33.
21. Follette VM, Pistorello J. Couples therapy. In: Classen C, Yalom ID, Classen C, Yalom ID (Eds). Treating women molested in childhood (pp. 129-161). Philadelphia: Jossey-Bass Publishers; 1995.
22. Forbes MK, Baillie AJ, Eaton NR, Krueger RF. (2017). A Place for
23. Fox KCR, Nijeboer S, Dixon ML, Floman JL, Ellamil M, Rumak SP, et al. Is meditation associated with altered brain structure? A systematic review and meta-analysis of morphometric neuroimaging in meditation practitioners. Neurosci Biobehav Rev. 2014;43:48-73.
24. Frühauf S, Gerger H, Schmidt H, Munder M, Barth T. Efficacy of Psychological Interventions for Sexual Dysfunction: A Systematic Review and Meta-Analysis. Arch Sex Behav. 2013;42(6):915-33.
25. Gu J, Strauss C, Bond R, Cavanagh K. How do mindfulness-based cognitive therapy and mindfulness-based stress reduction improve mental health and wellbeing? A systematic review and meta-analysis of mediation studies. Clin Psychol Rev. 2015;37:1-12.
26. Gunzler C, Berner MM. Efficacy of psychosocial interventions in men and women with sexual dysfunctions—a systematic review of controlled clinical trials: Part 2. J Sex Med. 2012;9(12):3108-25.
27. Mindfulness-based group therapy for women with provoked vestibulodynia. [online] Available from https://med-fom-brotto.sites.olt.ubc.ca/files/2014/11/Brotto-et-al.-2015-Mindfulness-based-group-therapy-for-women-with-PVD-3016.pdf [Last accessed January, 2026].
28. Sexual Dysfunctions in an Empirical Taxonomy of Psychopathology. J Sex Res. 2017;54(4-5):465-85.